Minimally Invasive Oncologic Surgery, Part I

Editors

CLAUDIUS CONRAD
JAMES W. FLESHMAN Jr

SURGICAL ONCOLOGY CLINICS OF NORTH AMERICA

www.surgonc.theclinics.com

Consulting Editor
TIMOTHY M. PAWLIK

January 2019 • Volume 28 • Number 1

ELSEVIER

1600 John F. Kennedy Boulevard • Suite 1800 • Philadelphia, Pennsylvania, 19103-2899

http://www.theclinics.com

SURGICAL ONCOLOGY CLINICS OF NORTH AMERICA Volume 28, Number 1
January 2019 ISSN 1055-3207, ISBN-13: 978-0-323-65505-7

Editor: John Vassallo (j.vassallo@elsevier.com)
Developmental Editor: Sara Watkins

Surgical Oncology Clinics of North America (ISSN 1055-3207) is published quarterly by Elsevier Inc., 360 Park Avenue South, New York, NY 10010-1710. Months of publication are January, April, July, and October. Business and Editorial Offices: 1600 John F. Kennedy Blvd., Ste. 1800, Philadelphia, PA 19103-2899. Customer Service Office: 3251 Riverport Lane, Maryland Heights, MO 63043. Periodicals postage paid at New York, NY and additional mailing offices. Subscription prices are $306.00 per year (US individuals), $533.00 (US institutions) $100.00 (US student/resident), $352.00 (Canadian individuals), $674.00 (Canadian institutions), $205.00 (Canadian student/resident), $422.00 (foreign individuals), $674.00 (foreign institutions), and $205.00 (foreign student/resident). Foreign air speed delivery is included in all *Clinics* subscription prices. All prices are subject to change without notice. **POSTMASTER**: Send address changes to *Surgical Oncology Clinics of North America*, Elsevier Health Science Division, Subscription Customer Service, 3251 Riverport Lane, Maryland Heights, MO 63043. **Customer Service: 1-800-654-2452 (US and Canada). 314-447-8871 (outside US and Canada). Fax: 314-447-8029. E-mail: journalscustomerservice-usa@elsevier.com (for print support); journalsonline support-usa@elsevier.com (for online support)**.

Reprints. For copies of 100 or more, of articles in this publication, please contact the Commercial Reprints Department, Elsevier Inc., 360 Park Avenue South, New York, New York 10010-1710. Tel. 212-633-3874; Fax: 212-633-3820; E-mail: reprints@elsevier.com.

Surgical Oncology Clinics of North America is covered in *MEDLINE/PubMed (Index Medicus)* and *EMBASE/ Excerpta Medica, Current Contents/Clinical Medicine, and ISI/BIOMED.*

Contributors

CONSULTING EDITOR

TIMOTHY M. PAWLIK, MD, MPH, PhD, FACS, FRACS (Hon.)
Professor and Chair, Department of Surgery, The Urban Meyer III and Shelley Meyer
Chair for Cancer Research, Professor of Surgery, Oncology, and Health Services
Management and Policy, Surgeon in Chief, The Ohio State University Wexner Medical
Center, Columbus, Ohio, USA

EDITORS

CLAUDIUS CONRAD, MD, PhD, FACS
Chief of General Surgery and Surgical Oncology, Director, Hepato-Pancreato-Biliary
Surgery Saint Elizabeth's Medical Center, Tufts University School of Medicine, Boston,
MA, USA

JAMES W. FLESHMAN Jr, MD
Sparkman Endowed Chair in Surgery, Baylor University Medical Center, Professor of
Surgery, Texas A&M Health Science Center, Texas A&M University, Dallas, Texas, USA

AUTHORS

OSMAN AHMED, MD
Department of Gastroenterology and Hepatology, The University of Texas MD Anderson
Cancer Center, Houston, Texas, USA

ADNAN ALSEIDI, MD, EdM, FACS
Director, HPB Fellowship, Assoc. PD, General Surgery, Simulation Director, HPB
and Endocrine Surgery, Virginia Mason Medical Center, Seattle, Washington,
USA

INNE H.M. BOREL RINKES, MD, PhD
Department of Surgery, University Medical Center, Utrecht Cancer Center, Utrecht
University, Utrecht, The Netherlands

FRANSISCO BORJA DE LACY, MD
Department of Gastrointestinal Surgery, ICMDM, AIS Channel, Hospital Clínic, Barcelona,
Spain

JULIETTA CHANG, MD
Department of Surgery, Massachusetts General Hospital, Boston, Massachusetts,
USA

EMILY R. CHRISTISON-LAGAY, MD
Assistant Professor of Pediatric Surgery, Yale School of Medicine, New Haven,
Connecticut, USA

JORDAN M. CLOYD, MD
Assistant Professor, Department of Surgery, The Ohio State University, Columbus, Ohio, USA

NOAH A. COHEN, MD
Complex General Surgical Oncology Fellow, Memorial Sloan Kettering Cancer Center, New York, New York, USA

ANDREY FINEGERSH, MD
Resident, Division of Head and Neck Surgery, University of California, San Diego, San Diego, California, USA

YUMAN FONG, MD
Department of Surgery, City of Hope National Medical Center, Duarte, California, USA

NEIL D. GROSS, MD
Professor, Department of Head and Neck Surgery, The University of Texas MD Anderson Cancer Center, Houston, Texas, USA

JEROEN HAGENDOORN, MD, PhD
Department of Surgery, University Medical Center, Utrecht Cancer Center, Utrecht University, Utrecht, The Netherlands

FLOYD CHRISTOPHER HOLSINGER, MD
Professor, Division of Head and Neck Surgery, Stanford University, Palo Alto, California, USA

TAKEAKI ISHIZAWA, MD, PhD, FACS
Department of Gastroenterological Surgery, Cancer Institute Hospital, Japanese Foundation for Cancer Research, Tokyo, Japan

THOMAS PETER KINGHAM, MD
Associate Attending, Hepatopancreatobiliary Service, Department of Surgery, Director of Global Cancer Disparity Initiatives, Memorial Sloan Kettering Cancer Center, Associate Professor, Department of Surgery, Weill Cornell Medical College, New York, New York, USA

ANTONIO M. LACY, MD, PhD, FASCRS (Hon)
Department of Gastrointestinal Surgery, ICMDM, IDIBAPS, CIBEREHD, Hospital Clínic, Universitat de Barcelona, Barcelona, Spain

ALFONSO LAPERGOLA, MD
IRCAD, Research Institute Against Cancer of the Digestive System, Strasbourg, France

JEFFREY H. LEE, MD, MPH
Medical Director of Endoscopy, Director of Advanced Endoscopy Fellowship, Professor, Department of Gastroenterology and Hepatology, The University of Texas MD Anderson Cancer Center, Houston, Texas, USA

JACQUES MARESCAUX, MD, FACS, (Hon) FRCS, (Hon) FJSES
IHU-Strasbourg, Institute of Image-Guided Surgery, IRCAD, Research Institute Against Cancer of the Digestive System, Strasbourg, France

IZAAK QUINTUS MOLENAAR, MD, PhD
Department of Surgery, University Medical Center, Utrecht Cancer Center, Utrecht University, Utrecht, The Netherlands

DIDIER MUTTER, MD, PhD, FACS
Department of General, Digestive and Endocrine Surgery, University Hospital of Strasbourg, Strasbourg, France

CAROLIJN L.M.A. NOTA, BSc
Department of Surgery, City of Hope National Medical Center, Duarte, California, USA; Department of Surgery, University Medical Center, Utrecht Cancer Center, Utrecht University, Utrecht, The Netherlands

RYAN K. OROSCO, MD
Assistant Professor, Division of Head and Neck Surgery, Head and Neck Surgical Oncology, Moores Cancer Center, University of California, San Diego, San Diego, California, USA

PATRICK PESSAUX, MD, PhD
IHU-Strasbourg, Institute of Image-Guided Surgery, IRCAD, Research Institute Against Cancer of the Digestive System, Department of General, Digestive and Endocrine Surgery, University Hospital of Strasbourg, Strasbourg, France

GIUSEPPE QUERO, MD
IHU-Strasbourg, Institute of Image-Guided Surgery, Strasbourg, France

DAVID W. RATTNER, MD
Department of Surgery, Massachusetts General Hospital, Boston, Massachusetts, USA

JANELLE F. REKMAN, MD, MAEd, FRCSC
HPB Clinical Fellow, Virginia Mason Medical Center, Seattle, Washington, USA

AKIO SAIURA, MD, PhD
Department of Gastroenterological Surgery, Cancer Institute Hospital, Japanese Foundation for Cancer Research, Tokyo, Japan

FRANCINA JASMIJN SMITS, MD
Department of Surgery, University Medical Center, Utrecht Cancer Center, Utrecht University, Utrecht, The Netherlands

LUC SOLER, PhD
IRCAD, Research Institute Against Cancer of the Digestive System, Strasbourg, France

DANIEL THOMAS, MD
Department of Surgery, Yale School of Medicine, New Haven, Connecticut, USA

SILVIA VALVERDE, MD
Department of Gastrointestinal Surgery, ICMDM, AIS Channel, Hospital Clínic, Barcelona, Spain

YANGHEE WOO, MD
Department of Surgery, City of Hope National Medical Center, Duarte, California, USA

Contents

> Introduction of the fiberoptic light-source and CCD chip camera resulted in the rapid growth of minimally invasive surgical procedures. In surgical oncology, the change came slowly owing to concerns about adhering to oncological principals while learning to use new technology. Pioneers in minimally invasive colorectal surgery proved that minimally invasive resection for cancer was oncologically noninferior to traditional surgery. Early adopters treating esophageal and gastric cancer established that a minimally invasive approach was feasible with lower morbidity and equivalent oncologic outcomes. These results provide a basis for the extension of minimally invasive surgical techniques to other types of cancer surgery.

> The surgical oncologist of the future requires training in minimally invasive techniques. Increasing constraints on time and resources have led to a new emphasis on finding innovative ways to teach these surgical skills inside and outside the operating room. The goal of producing technically gifted minimally invasive surgical (MIS) oncologists requires robust, educationally sound training curricula. This article describes how MIS oncology training occurs at present with an outline of educational ideals training programs can strive for, provides two examples of successful MIS oncology programs to highlight effective strategies for moving forward, and introduces three new developments on the horizon.

> Virtual reality (VR) and augmented reality (AR) in complex surgery are evolving technologies enabling improved preoperative planning and intraoperative navigation. The basis of these technologies is a computer-based generation of a patient-specific 3-dimensional model from Digital Imaging and Communications in Medicine (DICOM) data. This article provides a state-of-the- art overview on the clinical use of this technology with a specific focus on hepatic surgery. Although VR and AR are still in an evolving stage with only some clinical application today, these technologies have

This article demonstrates surgical techniques of intraoperative fluorescence imaging using indocyanine green, focusing on its application in minimally invasive hepatobiliary and pancreatic surgery. In this area, indocyanine green fluorescence imaging has been applied to liver cancer identification, fluorescence cholangiography, delineation of hepatic segments, and fluorescence angiography and perfusion assessment. The development of target-specific fluorophores and advances in imaging technology will allow real-time intraoperative fluorescence imaging to develop into an essential intraoperative navigation tool. This property may contribute to enhancing both accuracy and safety of minimally invasive surgery.

Staging laparoscopy (SL) is used to assess for radiographically occult metastatic disease and local resectability in selected patients with gastrointestinal malignancies. SL may avoid nontherapeutic laparotomy in patients with unresectable cancer and is associated with shorter length of hospital stay and time to receipt of systemic therapy compared with nontherapeutic laparotomy. With improvements in preoperative imaging, careful patient selection for SL is imperative. SL and peritoneal washings should be considered for patients with distal gastroesophageal and locally advanced gastric cancer before planned neoadjuvant chemotherapy or resection. SL should be considered in selected high-risk patients with hepatopancreatobiliary malignancies.

Palliative care is the multidisciplinary focus on patient symptoms and quality of life. The emphasis of minimally invasive surgery on reduced pain and faster recovery aligns well with the goals of palliative care. Minimally invasive approaches can be safely and effectively used to address several common complications of solid organ malignancies as well as the complications of cytotoxic therapy. A patient-centered, minimally invasive approach will not only help alleviate disabling symptoms and improve patient quality of life but will also minimize the pain and adverse effects of the intervention itself.

Indications for robotic surgery have been rapidly expanding since the first introduction of the robotic surgical system in the US market in 2000. As the robotic systems have become more sophisticated over the past decades, there has been an expansion in indications. Many new tools have been added with the aim of optimizing outcomes after oncologic surgery. Complex abdominal cancers are increasingly operated on using robot-assisted laparoscopy and with acceptable outcomes. In this article, the authors discuss robotic developments, from the past and the future, with an emphasis on cancer surgery.

Transluminal surgery, also known as natural orifices endoluminal surgery, can be considered the most minimally invasive approach of gaining access to an organ. Although some approaches, such as transgastric or transvaginal cholecystectomy, have remained experimental, peroral endoscopic myotomy to treat achalasia and transanal total mesorectal excision to treat low rectal cancer have become accepted, safe, and feasible approaches by trained surgeons for selected patients. This article recapitulates the development of transluminal surgery from its experimental beginnings to the validated procedure it has become today.

Robotic head and neck surgery applies minimally invasive principles to unique anatomy and natural orifices for surgical access. Expanding from a tradition of minimally invasive endoscopic otolaryngology procedures, surgical robotics has transformed head and neck surgery. However, surgeons are faced with significant challenges, and anatomic constraints impede visualization and constrain surgical maneuvers. Transoral robotic surgery (TORS) has been developed over the past decade with favorable oncologic and functional outcomes, changing the way head and neck surgeons approach both malignant and benign diseases. As new robotic platforms emerge, access will continue to improve and push the boundaries of minimally invasive approaches.

Over the last decade, driven in part by the favorable adult experience and a crescendoing number of case series and retrospective reports in the pediatric surgical literature, minimally invasive surgical (MIS) approaches are increasingly used as adjunctive or definitive surgical treatments for an ever-expanding list of pediatric tumors. Although most current treatment protocols lack surgical guidelines regarding the use of MIS, this growing body of MIS literature provides a framework for the development of multicenter trial groups, prospective registries, and further centralization of subspecialist services. This article highlights the current available data on MIS approaches to a variety of pediatric malignancies.

The role of endoscopy in the care of patients with pancreatic cancer continues to evolve. The early diagnosis of pancreatic cancer has been difficult. Endoscopic ultrasound examination should be used to examine pancreatic lesions because it can characterize lesions and sample tissue. Endoscopic retrograde cholangiopancreatography is essential in managing biliary obstructions. Endoscopic ultrasound can assist in gaining access to difficult biliary trees. Endoscopic placement of luminal stents can be used for palliative purposes. Postoperative issues such as strictures and anastomotic ulcers can generally be managed endoscopically. Injectable therapy and drug-eluting stent placements are potential areas for use in the future.

SURGICAL ONCOLOGY
CLINICS OF NORTH AMERICA

SERIES OF RELATED INTEREST

Surgical Clinics of North America
http://www.surgical.theclinics.com
Thoracic Surgery Clinics
http://www.thoracic.theclinics.com
Advances in Surgery
http://www.advancessurgery.com

THE CLINICS ARE AVAILABLE ONLINE!
Access your subscription at:
www.theclinics.com

Foreword
Minimally Invasive Oncologic Surgery

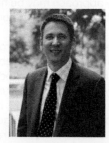

Timothy M. Pawlik, MD, MPH, PhD, FACS, RACS (Hon.)
Consulting Editor

This issue of *Surgical Oncology Clinics of North America* is devoted to advances and innovations in the surgical techniques around oncologic surgery. Over the past two decades there has been a dramatic increase in the interest and application of the minimally invasive approach to the management of cancer. The increase in utilization of the minimally invasive approach can be attributed to patient demand as well as data demonstrating improved perioperative outcomes associated with the minimally invasive approach compared with open surgery. For example, the minimally invasive approach has been associated with smaller incisions, less incisional pain, reduced need for opioids, shorter length of stay, as well as possibly lower overall morbidity and improved quality of life. The potential benefits of minimally invasive surgery, especially as they relate to patients with cancer, are several-fold. Surgery has long been thought of as a "stressor" with associated immunomodulation and possibly derivative effects on cancer progression. Many hypotheses exist regarding the immunologic response to surgery and whether a less "stressful" minimally invasive approach might result in better oncologic outcomes. Similarly, opioid use has been postulated by some to have a potential effect on angiogenesis and cellular-mediated immunity. As such, a minimally invasive approach that is more "opioid sparing" due to less associated incisional pain could theoretically benefit patients with cancer. While these topics remain debated and controversial, there are prospective data to suggest that the minimally invasive approach has at least comparable oncologic outcomes as open surgery. Specifically, the Clinical Outcomes of Surgical Therapy trial, which randomized 872 patients with colonic adenocarcinoma to open versus laparoscopically assisted colectomy, demonstrated the two groups were not significantly different in terms of local and overall survival at 3 years. Similarly, the European Colon Cancer Laparoscopic or Open Resection study group trial compared results for colon cancer between laparoscopic and open surgery. There also was no difference between the two groups with respect to morbidity and mortality. Taken together, the comparable oncologic outcomes combined with the improved perioperative patient-centered outcomes (eg, pain, length-of-stay, quality of life) make the minimally invasive approach to cancer surgery appealing. However, other studies have demonstrated that caution needs to be exercised. For example, one study on laparoscopic versus open resection for rectal cancer noted that laparoscopic surgery failed to meet the criterion for noninferiority for pathologic outcomes compared with open resection and thus was potentially inferior. As such, while enthusiasm for the minimally approach may be high, additional data and studies are needed to ensure comparable oncologic outcomes for some cancers/anatomic locations.

To address the important topic of minimally invasive oncologic surgery, I enlisted guest editors Claudius Conrad and James Fleshman from Saint Elizabeth's Medical Center and Baylor Scott and White, respectively. Both Dr Conrad and Dr Fleshman are well-recognized experts in the field of minimally invasive cancer surgery. Dr Conrad and Dr Fleshman have published extensively on this topic and have led trials examining the minimally invasive versus open approach for cancer surgery. In addition to their own expertise, Dr Conrad and Dr Fleshman enlisted a broad array of other experts in the field to put together a fantastic, comprehensive review.

This is a wonderful, comprehensive, and thorough state-of-the-art review on a wide range of topics pertaining to minimally invasive oncologic surgery that will be very relevant to all practicing surgical oncologists. I would like to thank Dr Conrad and Dr Fleshman and their wonderful group of colleagues for an excellent issue of the *Surgical Oncology Clinics of North America* and in taking on such an important topic.

Timothy M. Pawlik, MD, MPH, PhD, FACS, RACS (Hon.)
Professor and Chair, Department of Surgery
The Urban Meyer III and Shelley Meyer Chair for Cancer Research
The Ohio State University
Wexner Medical Center
395 W. 12th Avenue, Suite 670
Columbus, OH 43210, USA

E-mail address:
tim.pawlik@osumc.edu

Preface

Minimally Invasive Oncologic Surgery, Part I

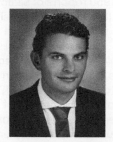
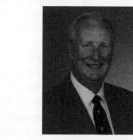

Claudius Conrad, MD, PhD, FACS   James W. Fleshman Jr, MD
Editors

*The secret of change is to focus all of your energy not on fighting the old, but on
building the new.*
—*Socrates in Way of the Peaceful Warrior, Dan Millman, 1980*

The history of cancer is the story of human innovation. Since its earliest documentation
on papyrus in 1600 BC, possibly based on text fragments as old as 2500 BC, this so-
called emperor of maladies has challenged our ability to describe, understand, and
treat a disease.

Early attempts to physically describe cancer came from thinkers like Hippocrates
(460-370 BC), who termed tumors karkinos, Greek for crab, based on the visual effect
of its cut surface filled with "veins stretched on all sides as the crab has its feet." Later,
the understanding that cancer has the tendency to recur became known to the Roman
physician Celsus (25 BC to 50 AD), who stated: "After excision, even when a scar has
formed, nonetheless the disease has returned."

The early days of a surgical solution to cancer saw pioneers like John Hunter, Astley
Cooper, and John Warren, who had to perform invasive operations quickly yet precisely given the lack general anesthesia until 1846. The next generation of surgeons,
Bilroth (Germany), Handley (England), and Halsted (United States), developed cancer-specific operations. Their work, along with the collective efforts of the multidisciplinary community, continues to push the boundaries of our understanding and
brings us to a new crossroad today.

Modern cancer surgery has the unique and unprecedented capacity to go beyond
technical aspects of removing the tumor, focusing simultaneously on the cancer's
biology and its morbidity. For example, while Halsted's radical mastectomy
certainly helped many patients suffering from breast cancer, later attempts to

Surg Oncol Clin N Am 28 (2019) xv–xvii
https://doi.org/10.1016/j.soc.2018.08.004
1055-3207/19/© 2018 Published by Elsevier Inc.

reduce the morbidity in the context of progress in oncologic management led to a significant reduction of morbidity. Similarly, once surgeons such as Codivilla (1898), Kausch (1912), and Whipple (1935) pioneered the complex operation of a pancreaticoduodenectomy, attempts to perform the operation less invasively led to Gagner and Pomp reporting the first laparoscopic pancreaticoduodenectomy in 1994. In parallel, after the first successful liver resection by the German surgeon Langenbuch in 1888 (the specimen showed normal liver), the eagerness of performing liver surgery according to anatomic principles resulted in post-1950 reports of selective anatomic liver resection by Honjo (Japan), Lortat-Jacob (France), and Ton That Tung (Vietnam). Then, minimally invasive liver resection was introduced in the 1990s.

Like many daring innovations, early attempts to develop minimally invasive surgery have not always drawn praise, or even approval. For example, after Semm performed the first laparoscopic appendectomy from the gynecological clinic of Kiel in 1981, the president of the German Surgical Society wrote to the Board of Directors of the German Gynecological Society requesting suspension of Semm from medical practice. Stories of such challenging environments are numerous and well known, and the ability of surgeons to push through those have paved the way for the exciting time in cancer surgery we live in today. This historic time includes standardizing minimally invasive operations and augmenting its potential by injecting high-tech applications, such as augmented reality or fluorescent-guided surgery.

This issue of *Surgical Oncology Clinics of North America* on Minimally Invasive Cancer Management, written by experts from around the world, provides an up-to-date overview on the tremendous progress that has been made in this field. In my role as Editor, I was fortunate to learn about the frontiers of our field from the editorial process and from scientific exchange with the contributing authors. Reviewing the beautiful and concise articles summarizing the tremendous progress in the field of minimally invasive cancer surgery takes me back to early days in my career, at the threshold of committing to surgery as my specialty. Some of my professors discouraged me, envisioning that cancer surgery would have been completely replaced by the progress in systemic therapies by now. Reality has proven the opposite, where the efficacy of systemic therapies has allowed surgical interventions against cancer to become more aggressive and effective. I am humbled and honored to contribute to the community of minimally invasive surgeons who hope to help their patients' battles by skillfully trading morbidity for radical oncologic surgery, maximizing the time and quality of a patient's life with their loved ones.

This special issue would not have been possible without a dedicated team working together. I would like to thank consulting editor Tim Pawlik for his tireless enthusiasm, my coeditor Jim Fleshman for supporting my editorial work, the Elsevier editorial team Sara Watkins and John Vassallo for their openness to create such a comprehensive issue, and Eduardo Vega for his creative assistance.

Claudius Conrad, MD, PhD, FACS
Saint Elizabeth's Medical Center
Tufts University School of Medicine
736 Cambridge Street
Brighton, MA 02135, USA

James W. Fleshman Jr, MD
Texas A&M Health Science Center
Department of Surgery
Baylor University Medical Center
3500 Gaston Avenue
1st Floor Roberts Hospital
Dallas, TX 75246, USA

E-mail addresses:
cconrad1@mdanderson.org (C. Conrad)
james.fleshman@bswhealth.org (J.W. Fleshman)

History of Minimally Invasive Surgical Oncology

Julietta Chang, MD, David W. Rattner, MD*

KEYWORDS

- Laparoscopy • Minimally invasive surgery • Surgical oncology • Colorectal surgery
- Surgical history

KEY POINTS

- Minimally invasive surgical techniques were first developed to treat benign conditions.
- Descriptions of port site metastases and inadequate lymph node harvest from early attempts to treat patients with cancer reinforced a sense of caution in the surgical oncology community.
- The COST trial clearly demonstrated that minimally invasive surgical approaches were noninferior to traditional surgery for treating colon cancer.
- With better surgical devices and an ever-increasing body of data showing the oncologic adequacy of minimally invasive surgical procedures, there is a shift in approach toward less invasive treatment of abdominal and thoracic malignancies.

HISTORY OF LAPAROSCOPY IN GENERAL SURGERY

The first recorded laparoscopic procedure was performed on a dog by Georg Kelling in Dresden in 1901. Kelling introduced a cystoscope directly through the abdominal wall to observe the effects of pneumoperitoneum and coined the approach "coelioscopy."[1] At the time, he postulated that, with "air-tamponade," one might be able to stop hemorrhage from gastrointestinal bleeding, a condition that at the time carried a high mortality even with laparotomy. He wanted to observe the effects of pneumoperitoneum and used insufflation pressures as high as 100 mm Hg in his canine subjects. He observed that the intraabdominal organs seemed to be blanched and contracted, not unusual considering his insufflation pressures, but 18 of 20 dogs survived their diagnostic laparoscopies and recovered without any apparent ill effects. In 1910, Hans Christian Jacobaeus in Sweden was the first to report on his experience with placing cystoscopes into human peritoneal and thoracic cavities. This was done without pneumoperitoneum, and he termed his technique "laparothorascopy," from

Disclosure Statement: Dr D.W. Rattner has a consulting relationship with Olympus America.
Department of Surgery, Massachusetts General Hospital, 15 Parkman Street WACC 460, Boston, MA 02114, USA
* Corresponding author.
E-mail address: drattner@mgh.harvard.edu

the Greek *laparo*, meaning the soft space between the ribs and the hips, and *scopie*, to visualize.[1–3]

For decades afterward, laparoscopy was rarely used owing to limits in light conduction and telescopic visualization. The development of the fiberoptic light source and Hopkins rod-lens system in the 1960s revolutionized laparoscopic surgery, allowing for brighter, better images.[2] Laparoscopy was adopted earliest in gynecology, where laparoscopic-aided bipolar electrocoagulation was used for tubal ligation in the 1970s; laparoscopy was also used to diagnose ectopic pregnancies and retrieve oocytes for in vitro fertilization. General surgeons, however, were slow to adopt this new technology because visualization of the abdominal cavity was still limited to the individual holding the laparoscope. The introduction of the CCD chip camera mounted to the laparoscope in 1986 allowed all members of the surgical team to see the operative field and, therefore, participate in the operation. Enabled by videolaparoscopy, the field of minimally invasive surgery took off.[2]

Laparoscopic cholecystectomy was first introduced in the United States in 1988. A few short years later in 1991, it was declared the standard of care for cholecystectomies.[4] From 1988 to 1997, the proportion of elective cholecystectomies performed laparoscopically skyrocketed from 2.5% to 76.6%.[5] Although initially there was little evidence to demonstrate that laparoscopic surgery was as safe as open cholecystectomy in the treatment of benign gallbladder disease, the benefits were undeniable to patients and clinicians. The minimally invasive approach clearly decreased postoperative pain, pulmonary and wound complications, and duration of hospital stay. Studies comparing laparoscopic and open appendectomies followed, with metaanalyses demonstrating the laparoscopic approach to be associated with decreased duration of stay, postoperative pain, and wound morbidity.[6] Similarly, in foregut surgery, specifically Nissen fundoplication for reflux disease and Heller myotomy for achalasia, the laparoscopic approach was rapidly adopted because there was superior visualization of the target anatomy in addition to the advantages of minimally invasive access.[7]

LAPAROSCOPY IN SURGICAL ONCOLOGY

Although laparoscopic cholecystectomy was the first widely adopted minimally invasive general surgery procedure, diagnostic laparoscopy had been used to stage malignancy for more than a decade longer. As early as 1971, DeVita and colleagues[8] reported performing diagnostic peritoneoscopies on 38 patients with Hodgkin's disease to stage patients before the initiation of radiation therapy. These procedures were performed under local anesthesia and the patients were discharged home the following day after having avoided the morbidity of a laparotomy. DeVita and associates found that peritoneoscopy could more accurately stage both liver and splenic involvement compared with physical examination or abnormal laboratory values. In this series, patients tended to be upstaged owing to liver and splenic involvement after their diagnostic laparoscopy, which of course had significant clinical implications because this change necessitated the addition of chemotherapy in addition to radiation therapy.

In 1978, Cuschieri and colleagues[9] reported their experience using laparoscopy in 23 patients suspected of having pancreatic cancer. This study demonstrated the feasibility of the technology in obtaining tissue for histopathologic diagnosis as well as diagnostic cholangiography (endoscopic cholangiography was not yet widely adopted). In patients diagnosed with metastatic disease via laparoscopy, avoiding the morbidity of a laparotomy was clearly beneficial. Diagnostic laparoscopy was also used in the early era to diagnose other intraabdominal malignancies such as colon cancer, hepatocellular carcinoma, and metastatic spread from these and other malignancies.[10,11] The next milestone in laparoscopic staging of malignancy was the introduction of laparoscopic ultrasound examination. This adjunct significantly enhanced the yield of staging laparoscopy.[12] Starting in 1993, laparoscopic ultrasound examination was combining with diagnostic laparoscopy at some centers to increase the accuracy of staging intraabdominal malignancies, including gastroesophageal junction tumors, hepatocellular carcinomas, biliary tract cancers, and pancreatic adenocarcinomas.[13] Depending on the type of cancer, diagnostic laparoscopy with ultrasound examination was able to prevent futile laparotomy by changing the preoperative stage of the cancer in 5% to 55% of patients.[13]

The adoption of therapeutic laparoscopic procedures developed more slowly. This lag was in part related to the lack of devices that provided reliable hemostasis, the difficulty of mastering intracorporeal suturing and advanced laparoscopic surgical techniques, and the complexity of performing resections that respected established oncologic principles. Although the first laparoscopic colectomies were reported in 1991, there was a reluctance to use laparoscopic techniques to treat colorectal cancer. By 2007, even after randomized trials demonstrated that patients who underwent laparoscopic colon resection had equivalent disease-free outcomes compared with their laparotomy counterparts,[14] fewer than 6% of colorectal resections for cancer were reported to be performed laparoscopically.[15] This outcome may have been due to specific oncologic concerns that are reviewed elsewhere in this article. However, some of this may have been in part owing to the "bigger is better" surgical dictum that seemed to persist longer in the field of surgical oncology[16] than other domains of general surgery.

KEY CONCERNS IN THE ADOPTION OF LAPAROSCOPY IN SURGICAL ONCOLOGY
Port Site Metastases

In the early 1990s, sporadic case reports surfaced describing cases of straightforward laparoscopic cholecystectomy in patients with cholelithiasis who were found to have unsuspected adenocarcinoma of the gallbladder on postoperative pathology and then rapidly developed port site metastases. This finding raised concerns about seeding tumor at both the extraction site and other trocar sites.[17] Similar reports followed with the adoption of laparoscopic colectomy. For example, in a series of 14 patients with colon cancer reported in 1994, 3 patients developed port site metastases after laparoscopic colectomy, 2 through the extraction site and 1 at a remote trocar site. The authors postulated that this was due to increased manipulation of the tumor through a smaller extraction site, although this supposition does not account for the metastasis at the distant trocar site.[18] This report was followed by a strongly worded review in 1996 looking at 35 cases of port site recurrences after laparoscopic resection of colorectal cancer; 23 cases of recurrence after thorascopic resection of lung neoplasm, 12 cases of recurrence after laparoscopic cholecystectomy for incidentally discovered gallbladder carcinoma, and 10 cases after laparoscopic oophorectomy for ovarian cancer.[19] However, at least one-half of the cases of ovarian malignancy had gross evidence of peritoneal seeding at time of resection. The thorascopic cases included 2 cases of metastatic disease (endometrial cancer and sarcoma), and thus the occurrences of port side metastasis were likely more a marker of disease activity than a result of surgical technique. However, these concerns persisted.

Adequacy of Surgical Resection

In early descriptions of laparoscopic left hemicolectomy, there were concerns about the adequacy of high vascular ligation or lack thereof.[20] In addition, in case reports of laparoscopic colectomies, lymph node retrieval was not necessarily reported, raising alarm in the community about the oncologic adequacy of the resection performed. However, these fears were not borne out in published histopathologic studies of the early 1990s, which reported proximal and distal margins of resection as well as lymph node retrieval that compared favorably with institutional standards regarding open resection.[21,22] Hence, this concern was felt to be surgeon related rather than inherently attributable to the minimally invasive approach.

Effect of Pneumoperitoneum on Tumor Spread

In the early era of operative laparoscopy, there was concern that increased intraabdominal pressure during pneumoperitoneum and circulating air flow from insufflation could contribute to the spread of tumor cells during resection of tumors. Mouse models studying the spread of gastric cancer cells and the effect of pneumoperitoneum raised concern that tumor cells could seed sites of tissue injury, specifically port sites.[23] Subsequent studies in animal models, however, demonstrated no increased risk of tumor spread or metastatic disease with CO_2 insufflation compared with laparotomy in rat models with colon cancer.[24]

ADOPTION OF MINIMALLY INVASIVE SURGERY IN COLORECTAL CANCER

Owing to the numerous concerns raised about the oncologic adequacy of laparoscopic resection in colorectal cancer, a multicenter national noninferiority trial was initiated in 1994 and published in 2004. More than 800 patients were randomly assigned to undergo laparoscopic-assisted or open colon resection by carefully credentialed surgeons in the Clinical Outcomes of Surgical Therapy Study Group trial (COST trial).[14] The primary outcome was time to tumor recurrence. Laparoscopic resection was associated with significantly longer operative time (150 minutes vs 95 minutes), but with decreased duration of hospital stay and less parenteral narcotic and oral analgesic use. There was no significant difference in the adequacy of resection margins or lymphadenectomy between the groups. Intraoperative and postoperative complications, need for reoperation, and readmission rate were similar between the groups as well. Most important, there was no significant difference in the cumulative incidence of cancer recurrence between patients treated with laparoscopic resection compared with laparotomy nor was there a difference in overall or disease-free survival. There were 3 patients with tumor recurrence in their surgical wounds: 2 in the laparoscopy group and 1 in the laparotomy group. This result was not significantly different, allaying concerns about wound and trocar site metastases.

Another important study, the Conventional versus Laparoscopic-Assisted Surgery in Patients with Colorectal Cancer (CLASICC) trial, was published the following year. This also included patients with rectal cancer. In the CLASSIC trial, there was an increased incidence of positive radial margin after laparoscopic low anterior resection for rectal cancer, but this did not translate into an increased incidence of local recurrence at 3 years and the laparoscopic and open techniques were otherwise oncologically equivalent.[25]

After this trial, there still seemed to be slow adoption of minimally invasive surgery to treat colorectal cancer. Robinson and colleagues[15] reported that, between 2005 and 2007, there was only a minimal increase in the number of colorectal cancer resections performed laparoscopically from 4.7% to 6.7% of cases. However, this was likely in part because of underreporting owing to the lack of *International Classification of Diseases* codes for laparoscopic colon resections and inaccurate coding for minimally invasive procedures.[26]

By October of 2008, a specific *International Classification of Diseases*, 9th edition, code for laparoscopic colectomy was introduced.[27] In a retrospective study examining elective colorectal procedures in Washington and Oregon, Kwon and colleagues[27] found that the number of laparoscopic colectomies performed for cancer had increased from 29.5% in 2005% to 38.4% in 2010. This study also found that wound infections and duration of hospital stay were shorter with laparoscopic colectomy and there was no difference in the adequacy of lymphadenectomy.

Subsequent randomized trials, most notably the Colorectal cancer Laparoscopic or Open Resection (COLOR II) trial for rectal cancer, demonstrated an equivalent radial resection margin with laparoscopic approach,[28] demonstrating that, in appropriately selected patients under the care of trained minimally invasive surgeons, both colon and rectal cancers can be approached laparoscopically with decreased perioperative complications and equivalent oncologic outcomes.

MINIMALLY INVASIVE SURGERY IN ESOPHAGEAL CANCER

The incidence of esophageal cancer, particularly of the lower esophagus and the gastroesophageal junction, is rapidly increasing in the United States. Between 1999 and 2008, the incidence of esophageal adenocarcinoma in Caucasian men and women increased by 2% per year, and at an even higher rate in Hispanic men at 2.8% per year.[29] Esophagectomy offers the only meaningful chance for cure for localized esophageal cancer, although outcomes remain poor with a 5-year survival of 15% to 25%.[30] Traditional open esophagectomy is associated with high rates of morbidity and mortality in large part owing to the cardiopulmonary stress associated with access.[31] Reports of perioperative complications are upwards of 70% and hospital mortality of 4% after transhiatal esophagectomy,[32] and 80% and 2.9% after transthoracic esophagectomy.[33,34] As such, it is an ideal surgery to approach minimally invasively to decrease morbidity, especially given that patients with esophageal carcinoma tend to be debilitated with weight loss and associated comorbid conditions.[31]

DePaula and colleagues[35] were the first to report a series of 12 patients with both benign and malignant disease treated with laparoscopic transhiatal esophagectomy. There was 1 conversion to laparotomy owing to a liver laceration. The mean duration of stay in the series was 7 days, which was shorter than the authors' historic hospital stay for open esophagectomy. There were no deaths in this series, although the 2 patients with cancer developed postoperative complications including anastomotic leak, which resolved with percutaneous drainage, and pleural effusion. The authors did not comment on the margin status or adequacy of lymphadenectomy in either patient.

Shortly thereafter, Swanstrom and Hansen[31] reported their experience with a series of 9 patients in 1997. The majority had gastroesophageal junction cancer, 2 had Barrett's esophagus, and 1 had a peptic stricture. All patients underwent a laparoscopic transhiatal esophagectomy with no conversions to open laparotomy. There were no anastomotic leaks or wound complications in this series. There were 2 deaths from metastatic disease but no evidence of local recurrence in patients with stage 3 and 4 disease. Again, the pathology of the resected specimens is not reported in this series.

The following year, Luketich and coworkers[36] reported the University of Pittsburgh group's experience with minimally invasive esophagectomy for both benign and malignant disease in 8 patients. There were 2 conversions to minilaparotomy to facilitate dissection of the esophagus in one and to help mature the gastric conduit in the second. There was 1 cervical anastomotic leak and 1 patient with delayed gastric emptying requiring pyloroplasty, but, most important, no mortality in this series.

Fourteen years later, his group reported on more than 1000 patients undergoing mini-mally invasive esophagectomy from 1996 to 2011.[30] The conversion rate to open sur-gery (either thorascopic or laparoscopic to thoracotomy or laparotomy, respectively) was 4.5% in this series. The 30-day mortality was low at 1.68% and there were no intraoperative mortalities. The incidence of major postoperative morbidity was 25%. The R0 resection rate was 98%, and the median number of lymph nodes retrieved was 21, similar to outcomes reported with open resections. These studies show that in experienced centers, minimally invasive esophagectomies can be performed safely with good oncologic outcomes and with lower morbidity and mortality than an open approach.

ADOPTION OF MINIMALLY INVASIVE SURGERY IN GASTRIC CANCER

Gastric cancer is the second most common cause of cancer-related death world-wide.[37] The incidence of gastric cancer varies geographically and is much higher in East Asia compared with the United States.[38] In Japan and Korea, where the inci-dence of gastric cancer is very high, upper endoscopy is recommended every 2 to 3 years starting at age 50 or 40, respectively.

With the implementation of screening programs, there was an increase in the detec-tion of early gastric cancer potentially amenable to minimally invasive resection. The first laparoscopic-assisted distal gastrectomy with Billroth I reconstruction was per-formed in 1991 in by Kitano and colleagues[39] for early gastric cancer. They later re-ported on 28 patients randomized to laparoscopic-assisted distal gastrectomy versus conventional laparotomy for distal gastric cancer.[40] Fourteen patients under-went laparoscopic-assisted distal gastrectomy without need for conversion; these pa-tients had better pain control compared with their laparotomy counterparts, less impairment of their pulmonary function, and, most important, similar R0 resection rates on final pathology. Subsequently, an ever-increasing percentage of gastrec-tomies have been performed laparoscopically in Japan, Korea, and China. However, adoption has been much slower in the United States. This lag is likely because the inci-dence of gastric cancer is much lower in most Western countries and, when diag-nosed, is usually more advanced. Because laparoscopic gastrectomy is a technically challenging operation with a steep learning curve, many surgeons cannot garner the volume of cases to gain proficiency.[41]

LAPAROSCOPIC SPLENECTOMY

Open splenectomy was first described in 1910.[42] Splenectomy for various indications traditionally was performed via a midline laparotomy or a left subcostal incision. The most common indication for elective splenectomy in the adult population is treatment for idiopathic thrombotic purpura (ITP).[42] There exist various other hematologic indica-tions for splenectomy, including staging for Hodgkin's disease, treatment of marginal zone lymphoma, or therapeutic splenectomy for hereditary spherocytosis in the pedi-atric population.[43] Owing to the morbidity associated with the open approach, various hematologic conditions associated with splenic disease, especially ITP, were tradi-tionally managed medically, with surgery reserved for severe disease refractory to therapy.

Laparoscopic splenectomy was first reported in France by Delaitre and Maignien in 1991.[44] The next year in the United States, Carroll and colleagues[45] reported a series of 3 patients who underwent laparoscopic splenectomy, 2 for Hodgkin's disease and 1 for ITP. One patient underwent conversion to a left subcostal incision for uncon-trolled hemorrhage; the other 2 were successfully completed laparoscopically, demonstrating the feasibility of this technique. Shortly thereafter, this group published on 16 patients who underwent laparoscopic splenectomy for a variety of pathologies, the most common being ITP.[46] Thirteen were completed laparoscopically and conversions occurred owing to uncontrolled hemorrhage early in the center's experience, illustrating that like in all other laparoscopic procedures, there is a significant learning curve. ITP especially is suited for laparoscopic approach, because it is not associated with splenomegaly and there are few concerns with specimen morcellation for extraction. As experience increased, however, laparoscopic splenectomy became the approach of choice for certain types of lymphoma and splenic masses. The introduction of the "hanging spleen" approach by Delaitre[47] in 1995 was a major technical advance that made the laparoscopic approach possible for larger spleens.

Laparoscopic splenectomy was adopted more slowly in the pediatric population, perhaps because children are quicker to recover from surgery in general, so the benefits of minimal access surgery are less pronounced. The first pediatric laparoscopic splenectomy was described in 1993,[48] and in 1998 Curran and colleagues[49] compared 7 patients who underwent laparoscopic splenectomy with 7 patients who underwent laparotomy. This group found that laparoscopic approach decreased postoperative pain and duration of hospital stay; the laparoscopic group enjoyed improved cosmesis. There was no difference in intraoperative blood loss between groups; however, there was an increase in operative time noted with laparoscopic approach. There were no conversions to laparotomy in this series, demonstrating the safety of this approach in the pediatric population.

SUMMARY

Minimally invasive surgical techniques have come a long way since the early days of diagnostic peritoneoscopies. Patients with cancer in the future will greatly benefit from the pioneering work of surgeons in the 1990s who introduced these techniques in the face of harsh criticism from their colleagues. Although the surgical oncology community was initially slow to adopt these techniques, pioneers and their disciples went on to accumulate sound data, showing that minimally invasive techniques provided equivalent or even superior outcomes compared with traditional surgical approaches. Diseases such as colon cancer, early gastric cancer, and esophageal cancer are now preferentially approached with minimally invasive surgery with decreased pain, lower wound infection rates, better postoperative pulmonary function and shorter recovery time compared with traditional laparotomy. The introduction of new surgical tools and digital information technologies will accelerate this trend and expand the preference for minimally invasive approach to many other cancer operations.

REFERENCES

1. Litynski GS. Laparoscopy–the early attempts: spotlighting Georg Kelling and Hans Christian Jacobaeus. JSLS 1997;1:83–5.
2. Lau WY, Leow CK, Li AK. History of endoscopic and laparosoopic surgery. World J Surg 1997;21:444–53.
3. Antoniou SA, Antoniou GA, Koutras C, et al. Endoscopy and laparoscopy: a historical aspect of medical terminology. Surg Endosc 2012;26:3650–4.
4. Pappas TN. Laparoscopic cholecystectomy: the standard of care for chronic and acute cholecystitis. Ann Med 1991;23:231.
5. Kemp JA, Zuckerman RS, Finlayson SRG. Trends in adoption of laparoscopic cholecystectomy in rural versus urban hospitals. J Am Coll Surg 2008;206:28–32.

6. Chung RS, Rowland DY, Li P, et al. A meta-analysis of randomized controlled trials of laparoscopic versus conventional appendectomy. Am J Surg 1999;177:250–6.
7. Cuschieri A. The spectrum of laparoscopic surgery. World J Surg 1992;16: 1089–97.
8. DeVita VT, Bagley CM, Goodell B, et al. Peritoneoscopy in the staging of Hodgkin's disease. Cancer Res 1971;31:1746–50.
9. Cuschieri A, Hall AW, Clark J. Value of laparoscopy in the diagnosis and management of pancreatic carcinoma. Gut 1978;19:672–7.
10. Easter DW, Cuschieri A, Nathanson LK, et al. The utility of diagnostic laparoscopy for abdominal disorders. Audit of 120 patients. Arch Surg 1992;127:379–83.
11. Cuschieri A. Role of video-laparoscopy in the staging of intra-abdominal lymphomas and gastrointestinal cancer. Semin Surg Oncol 2001;20:167–72.
12. Cuschieri A. Laparoscopic management of cancer patients. J R Coll Surg Edinb 1995;40:1–9.
13. Gouma DJ, de Wit LT, Nieveen van Dijkum E, et al. Laparoscopic ultrasonography for staging of gastrointestinal malignancy. Scand J Gastroenterol Suppl 1996; 218:43–9.
14. Clinical Outcomes of Surgical Therapy Study Group, Nelson H, Sargent DJ, Wieand HS, et al. A comparison of laparoscopically assisted and open colectomy for colon cancer. N Engl J Med 2004;350:2050–9.
15. Robinson CN, Chen GJ, Balentine CJ, et al. Minimally invasive surgery is underutilized for colon cancer. Ann Surg Oncol 2011;18:1412–8.
16. Pappas TN, Jacobs DO. Laparoscopic resection for colon cancer — the end of the beginning? N Engl J Med 2004;350:2091–2.
17. Wade TP, Comitalo JB, Andrus CH, et al. Laparoscopic cancer surgery. Lessons from gallbladder cancer. Surg Endosc 1994;8:698–701.
18. Berends FJ, Kazemier G, Bonjer HJ, et al. Subcutaneous metastases after laparoscopic colectomy. Lancet 1994;344:58.
19. Johnstone PA, Rohde DC, Swartz SE, et al. Port site recurrences after laparoscopic and thoracoscopic procedures in malignancy. J Clin Oncol 1996;14: 1950–6.
20. Milsom JW, Fazio VW. Concerns about laparoscopic colon cancer surgery. Dis Colon Rectum 1994;37:625–6.
21. Van Ye TM, Cattey RP, Henry LG. Laparoscopically assisted colon resections compare favorably with open technique. Surg Laparosc Endosc 1994;4:25–31.
22. Moore JW, Bokey EL, Newland RC, et al. Lymphovascular clearance in laparoscopically assisted right hemicolectomy is similar to open surgery. Aust N Z J Surg 1996;66:605–7.
23. Hirabayashi Y, Yamaguchi K, Shiraishi N, et al. Development of port-site metastasis after pneumoperitoneum. Surg Endosc 2002;16:864–8.
24. Tomita H, Marcello PW, Milsom JW, et al. CO2 pneumoperitoneum does not enhance tumor growth and metastasis: study of a rat cecal wall inoculation model. Dis Colon Rectum 2001;44:1297–301.
25. Jayne DG, Guillou PJ, Thorpe H, et al. Randomized trial of laparoscopic-assisted resection of colorectal carcinoma: 3-year results of the UK MRC CLASICC Trial Group. J Clin Oncol 2007;25:3061–8.
26. Wexner SD. Underutilization of minimally invasive surgery for colorectal cancer. Ann Surg Oncol 2011;18:1518–9.
27. Surgical Care and Outcomes Assessment Program (SCOAP) Collaborative, Kwon S, Billingham R, Farrokhi E, et al. Adoption of laparoscopy for elective

colorectal resection: a report from the Surgical Care and Outcomes Assessment Program. J Am Coll Surg 2012;214:909–18.e1.
28. van der Pas MH, Haglind E, Cuesta MA, et al. Laparoscopic versus open surgery for rectal cancer (COLOR II): short-term outcomes of a randomised, phase 3 trial. Lancet Oncol 2013;14:210–8.
29. Simard EP, Ward EM, Siegel R, et al. Cancers with increasing incidence trends in the United States: 1999 through 2008. CA Cancer J Clin 2012;62:118–28.
30. Luketich JD, Pennathur A, Awais O, et al. Outcomes after minimally invasive esophagectomy. Ann Surg 2012;256:95–103.
31. Swanstrom LL, Hansen P. Laparoscopic total esophagectomy. Arch Surg 1997; 132:943–7 [discussion: 947–9].
32. Orringer MB, Marshall B, Iannettoni MD. Transhiatal esophagectomy for treatment of benign and malignant esophageal disease. World J Surg 2001;25:196–203.
33. Goldfaden D, Orringer MB, Appelman HD, et al. Adenocarcinoma of the distal esophagus and gastric cardia. Comparison of results of transhiatal esophagectomy and thoracoabdominal esophagogastrectomy. J Thorac Cardiovasc Surg 1986;91:242–7.
34. Mathisen DJ, Grillo HC, Wilkins EW, et al. Transthoracic esophagectomy: a safe approach to carcinoma of the esophagus. Ann Thorac Surg 1988;45:137–43.
35. DePaula AL, Hashiba K, Ferreira EA, et al. Laparoscopic transhiatal esophagectomy with esophagogastroplasty. Surg Laparosc Endosc 1995;5:1–5.
36. Luketich JD, Nguyen NT, Weigel T, et al. Minimally invasive approach to esophagectomy. JSLS 1998;2:243–7.
37. Lambert R, Guilloux A, Oshima A, et al. Incidence and mortality from stomach cancer in Japan, Slovenia and the USA. Int J Cancer 2002;97:811–8.
38. Jemal A, Bray F, Center MM, et al. Global cancer statistics. CA Cancer J Clin 2011;61:69–90.
39. Kitano S, Iso Y, Moriyama M, et al. Laparoscopy-assisted Billroth I gastrectomy. Surg Laparosc Endosc 1994;4:146–8.
40. Kitano S, Shiraishi N, Uyama I, et al. A multicenter study on oncologic outcome of laparoscopic gastrectomy for early cancer in Japan. Ann Surg 2007;245:68–72.
41. Chang J, Kroh M. Robotic partial and total gastrectomy. SAGES Man. Robot. Surg. Cham (Switzerland): Springer International Publishing; 2018. p. 297–308.
42. Rosen M, Brody F, Walsh RM, et al. Outcome of laparoscopic splenectomy based on hematologic indication. Surg Endosc 2002;16:272–9.
43. Wilhelm MC, Jones RE, McGehee R, et al. Splenectomy in hematologic disorders. The ever-changing indications. Ann Surg 1988;207:581–9.
44. Delaitre B, Maignien B. Splenectomy by the laparoscopic approach. Report of a case. Presse Med 1991;20:2263 [in French].
45. Carroll BJ, Phillips EH, Semel CJ, et al. Laparoscopic splenectomy. Surg Endosc 1992;6:183–5.
46. Phillips EH, Carroll BJ, Fallas MJ. Laparoscopic splenectomy. Surg Endosc 1994; 8:931–3.
47. Delaitre B. Laparoscopic splenectomy. The "hanged spleen" technique. Surg Endosc 1995;9:528–9.
48. Tulman S, Holcomb GW, Karamanoukian HL, et al. Pediatric laparoscopic splenectomy. J Pediatr Surg 1993;28:689–92.
49. Curran TJ, Foley MI, Swanstrom LL, et al. Laparoscopy improves outcomes for pediatric splenectomy. J Pediatr Surg 1998;33:1498–500.

Training for Minimally Invasive Cancer Surgery

Janelle F. Rekman, MD, MAEd[a,b,*], Adnan Alseidi, MD, EdM[b,c]

KEYWORDS

- Minimally invasive surgery • Education • Training • Oncology • Fellowship
- Simulation

KEY POINTS

- Minimally invasive surgical (MIS) oncology training programs face three major challenges: rapid technology change and uptake, resource strain causing decreased trainee operative time, and promotion of excellent patient outcomes and oncologic quality.
- Various forms of simulated learning are taking precedence in MIS training programs. Validity and fidelity testing are ongoing for advanced laparoscopic skill training models.
- Current and future MIS training programs must incorporate proven curriculum development methodology if programs are to be increasingly effective and efficient.

INTRODUCTION

The surgical oncologist of the future must not only develop a deep understanding of cancer biology, but must also become technically proficient in open and minimally invasive techniques. Minimally invasive surgery (MIS) has moved beyond frontier research, becoming near standard of care for many oncologic procedures. With the rapid uptake of MIS techniques over a generation, there is pressure on the MIS trainee to quickly become the trainer.

Increasing constraints on time and resources required to train MIS oncologic surgeons have led to a new emphasis on finding innovative ways to teach surgical skills, inside and outside the operating room (OR). The sense of urgency to acquire MIS skills has spurred the development of many fellowship and short-course training programs, and a rapid advancement of training technology options. Since Frederich Greene told

Disclosure Statement: Dr J. Rekman has no financial, commercial, or funding disclosures. Dr A. Alseidi has no relevant financial, commercial, or funding disclosures; speaker, Ethicon Endosurgery.
[a] General Surgery, University of Ottawa, 427 Sunnyside Avenue, Apartment A, Ottawa, Ontario K1S0S6, Canada; [b] Virginia Mason Medical Center, 1100 Ninth Avenue, GS-C6, Seattle, WA 98101, USA; [c] HPB and Endocrine Surgery, Virginia Mason Medical Center, 1100 Ninth Avenue, GS-C6, Seattle, WA 98101, USA
* Corresponding author.
E-mail address: janelle.rekman@virginiamason.org

Surg Oncol Clin N Am 28 (2019) 11–30
https://doi.org/10.1016/j.soc.2018.07.007
1055-3207/19/© 2018 Elsevier Inc. All rights reserved.

the World Congress of Laparoscopic Surgery in 1998, "The capacity of American surgery to adequately teach advanced minimally invasive surgery is simply overwhelmed,"[1] how far has the field come?

Throughout the literature are exciting examples of how specialists and generalists alike are working to overcome the educational challenges of this rapid evolution. The Halstedian training model based on imitation and learning by doing formerly prepared surgeons for a lifelong static practice. This model is now stretching actively to accommodate technologic changes that force surgeons to retrain multiple times in the course of their career.

MIS training programs have the added burden of striving for excellent oncologic outcomes, in addition to the expected patient safety outcomes. In the hurry to train new MIS surgeons, the prize MIS surgical oncologists are striving for should be not only "can this be done?," but also, "is this oncologically appropriate?".

This article describes how MIS oncology training occurs at present with a quick outline of educational ideals training programs can strive for, highlights two examples of successful MIS oncology programs to show effective strategies for moving forward, and introduces three exciting new developments on the horizon.

CURRENT MINIMALLY INVASIVE SURGICAL ONCOLOGY TRAINING

Thirty years of laparoscopic surgical experience has led to a wealth of discussion regarding educational strategies for introducing new technology into training. Recently, this conversation has re-engaged, albeit from a slightly different angle, as robotics have entered mainstream practice. This discussion is occurring in two distinct arenas: structured training programs and continuing professional development. Decisions in one sphere affect the other, as staff surgeons learning new techniques exit the realm of trainer for a time until they are competent to return to structured programs. Those currently seeking MIS training, no matter what stage of practice, have multiple opportunities at their fingertips.

The complex nature of advanced MIS offers a unique challenge to medical educators. The Society of American Gastrointestinal Endoscopic Surgeons (SAGES) has recognized these concerns and issued several position papers and statements regarding resident training, practice safety, and credentialing standards for surgeons who wish to incorporate basic and advanced techniques into practice.[2] General surgery basic MIS procedures (according to SAGES) are: laparoscopic appendectomy, cholecystectomy, and diagnostic laparoscopy. All other laparoscopic procedures are defined as "advanced." Ideally, advanced MIS skills would be acquired during residency training, but there are numerous limitations on this goal.

The technical skills a minimally invasive surgical oncologist must demonstrate are grounded in solid basic maneuvers, such as the fulcrum effect of long, stick-like instruments working further away from you; hand-eye coordination; camera manipulation; clip application; and the transformation of the image on a two-dimensional monitor into actions in a three-dimensional workspace. These basic maneuvers pave the way to advanced techniques for achieving hemostasis, exposure of organs, and two-handed surgical manipulation and dissection. What the nondominant hand does in open surgery is not enough for laparoscopic surgery, where with constrained space and working angles it must take a more active role. And what one may "get away with" outside the correct surgical plane in open surgery, may spell conversion if one is not careful and deliberate in an advanced laparoscopic procedure. Movements that require large thought input at the beginning of a learning curve need to become automated so attention is focused on more sophisticated actions.

Although MIS oncology procedures are considered standard of care in many places, global uptake of MIS technique varies drastically. Even today in many Western training programs open surgery dominates training.[3] Trainees in programs still working to incorporate MIS into their repertoire struggle to gain advanced laparoscopic skill.[4]

CASE STUDY: THE INTRODUCTION OF LAPAROSCOPIC HEPATECTOMY

Understanding how laparoscopic hepatectomy is being introduced into mainstream surgical practice is a case study in the current challenges of advanced MIS training. The Second International Consensus Conference on Laparoscopic Liver Resection in Japan concluded that patients having laparoscopic liver surgery have fewer complications and equivalent outcomes.[5] However, this same conference proceeded to recommend cautious introduction of the technique into mainstream practice. Studies have shown that reproducing these positive outcomes comes only after a long learning curve of 60 cases.[5,6] Bleeding in this solid organ is challenging to control,[7] and strategies for troubleshooting are different than in open surgery.

If one believes in the benefits of laparoscopic liver resection, how then can laparoscopic hepatectomy training be disseminated? Trainees cannot be expected to teach themselves an advanced minimally invasive liver resection through online learning. At this point in time knowledgeable proctors who could take time away to mentor are few. There are no standardized simulators widely available to walk a surgeon through a minimally invasive hepatectomy, and developing them will be expensive and time-consuming.

Any solution needs to be accessible to residency trainees, and to surgeons looking to develop new skills in practice. As demonstrated by Yamada and colleagues[8] in the curriculum they have developed for MIS hepatectomy, it is through a multimodal approach, introduced in a stepwise and thoughtful fashion, that proficiency is achieved. Advanced MIS skill and judgment take time to mature, and as discussed later, there are programmatic ways to work to create effective MIS training programs.

SIMULATED LEARNING

Most residency programs are structured, with majority of MIS training beginning outside the OR, with the intent to transition to graded responsibility in the OR as skills and opportunity allow. Junior trainees observe or assist on procedures that they practice in the simulation laboratory and simulation models are abundant (inanimate, such as video, box, virtual reality [VR]; and animate, such as live animal or cadaver). Whether or not the simulation laboratory should be a substitute for in-OR learning is a well-oiled debate propelled by a range of considerations: public opinion and patient safety concerns, OR efficiency and economics, restricted resident work hours, and the increased technical requirements of MIS surgery itself. A surgical trainee can no longer "just try" in the OR as in the early days of open surgery.

BASIC SKILLS SIMULATION

The value of simulation for developing basic laparoscopic skills has been widely accepted. In the words of Dr. Gerald Fried, cocreator of the McGill Inanimate System for Training and Evaluation of Laparoscopic Skills (MISTELS), "I am tired of seeing people come into the OR and put their instruments right through the liver because they haven't yet learned cues for depth perception. Or their hands are all over the place because they are not used to the amplification of movement of an instrument placed through a trocar."[9] Many simulators have been developed for teaching basic MIS technical skills. Each training model has its relative advantages and disadvantages (**Table 1**), and several systematic reviews and double-blind randomized controlled trials (RCTs) have demonstrated acquisition of technical skill to occur effectively on all of these simulators.[10–12]

The focus of research in simulation for basic laparoscopic training has changed from examining whether it works, to how best to implement it. For example, manufacturing of affordable, portable box trainers for convenient anytime use at home can increase access to training. It is key, however, to ensure that repetitive off-site independent practice does not lead to development of bad habits. In addition, spreading experience out over time (distributed practice), rather than intense, multihour sessions (amassed practice) has been shown to improve retention.[13] Independent of where or when the simulated experience occurs, assessment by a trainer (immediately vs remotely) needs to occur for the trainee to have any benefit from the system.[14]

SIMULATION FOR ADVANCED MINIMALLY INVASIVE SURGERY SKILLS

What is not clear is the educational value resulting from simulation for advanced procedures, because of poor quality evidence.[15] Do advanced skills learned in a

Table 1
Relative advantages and disadvantages of simulated training models

Training Model	Advantages	Disadvantages
Box/mechanical trainers	• Practice "off-site" possible • Outside of training hours • "Distributed," rather than "amassed," practice • Cheap • Reproducible • Training of isolated skills • Standardized	• Low fidelity • Little to no tissue similarity
Virtual reality simulators	• Repetition of steps • Objective feedback from program • Performance of real operation	• Costly • Software and interface issues • Minimal haptic feedback
Animal and cadaver models	• Good tissue handling • Anatomic accuracy • No time pressure • Live animal models bleed	• Costly • Resource-intense • Ethically charged • Cadavers: noncompliant, bloodless tissues • Live animals: one-time use
Short courses	• Presence of many experts able to give "tips and tricks" • Time efficiency constrained • E-learning courses can be done from home, on own time	• "Amassed" practice • Limited evidence of incorporation of technique into practice
Peer mentoring and coaching	• Time for self-reflection • "Distributed" practice • Expert coaching eyes and ears in the room • Refining of advanced technical skills • Identification of previously unrecognized areas of improvement	• Being involved in a coaching program may be perceived as synonymous with incompetence • Can be costly • Explanation to patients requires assertion of nonperfection

simulated setting actually transfer to improved performance in the OR? The main tools used in advanced MIS training are pig models and virtual trainers involving animal organs (cheaper than synthetic models).[16] Whole-procedure models have also been tried.[17] Laparoscopic colorectal surgeons have created a programmatic approach for advanced laparoscopic colorectal MIS training, and even here only one RCT has shown transfer of advanced laparoscopic colorectal surgery (LCS) skills to the OR.[18] Despite, this much of the background framework-building research has been done in general surgery and does not need to be replicated,[19] and there is a wealth of research being performed in urology and gynecology MIS training programs.[20]

Virtual Reality Simulators

Outside of wet laboratories there are many options for VR simulation, especially with the advent of robotics. A recent Cochrane review showed VR technology improves laparoscopic skills in trainees with limited previous experience, compared with conventional training and with a box trainer.[11] Aggarwal and colleagues[21] took this a step further and showed that repetitive practice to proficiency on a VR laparoscopic cholecystectomy model shortens the learning curve for this basic MIS procedure in the OR.

Robotic simulators recently developed for the Da Vinci surgical system console demonstrate high-fidelity outcomes because the trainee is sitting at the same console that is used in the OR with identical instrumentation.[22] Despite the emphasis on VR simulation in robotic training, minimal strong evidence exists to date that it actually improves performance in the OR. In general, there is evidence that novice surgeons gain robotic and laparoscopic skills on VR simulators[23]; however, data on advanced skill acquisition are still being acquired as technology rapidly advances.

Fellowship Programs

In 1991 there were three MIS general surgery fellowships in the United States, in 1993 there were nine, and by 2004 there were 80.[24] Today there are more than 156 programs and 210 fellowship positions in specialty surgery ranging from endoscopy to MIS to Hepato Pancreato Biliary (HPB) to colorectal.[25] Originally, it was thought that as more MIS surgeons were trained, residency programs would take on the role fellowship programs once played. However, this does not seem to be occurring. In 2011, 70% to 80% of general surgery residents in North America sought further fellowship training.[26,27] Fellowship training is taking the role of advanced MIS training not occurring at the residency level and in a way, these fellowships are now becoming a requirement of hiring departments.

Short Courses

Most evidence supporting short courses for MIS training demonstrates their ability to increase knowledge base before being in the OR. Online courses taken on the trainee's own time without the need to travel are one option.[28] Online courses show numerous benefits compared with traditional didactic learning in that they can incorporate animations and demonstrations, are standardized, and do not require a proctor.[29,30] However, there is limited technical skill development potential.

Procedure-specific short courses including hands-on animal, cadaver, or live surgery courses are the most common examples of off-site training.[31] There is evidence to say that short courses using didactic training and animal models are out-done by directed intraoperative preceptorship, in terms of outcomes, conversion rate, and up-take (surgeons continuing to perform procedure using MIS technique in the future).[32] The main shortfall of these courses is lack of linkage between coursework outside of the trainee's institution with what actually happens in their OR.[33] **Table 2** provides a summary of other common pitfalls to be avoided when introducing and participating in short courses. In general short courses are a stepping-stone toward uptake of advanced MIS procedures into practice, but alone, they do not convey enough experience for a surgeon to become proficient in a procedure.[34] In addition, they are more beneficial to surgeons with advanced skill looking to pick up new techniques, not to brand new trainees (see **Table 2**).[35]

ONLINE VIDEOS

In the era of OR efficiency and an increasing number of fellows, resident observation time has increased. Although there is constant debate as to how much time trainees should spend observing versus actually practicing, studies show an intentional mix of both is complementary.[36] The benefits of using multimedia tools, including use of operative video recording, to catalyze the development of surgical skills are well known. Observing operative steps in video form converts cognitive input into long-term image memory more efficiently than just reading them.[37]

It is common now that videos be used to prepare for, and review, operative cases. With high-definition recordings of MIS procedures easily accessed from the couch at home, this potential major learning resource requires attention. Mota and colleagues[38] found that young surgical trainees prefer to use online resources narrated with voice-over walking them through the steps. In contrast, staff surgeons value the technical

Table 2	
Common pitfalls of MIS short courses	
No proctor knowledge of trainee needs	• It is important to begin where the learners are at, not where you were planning to • A short set of precourse questions and consideration of example video submission could provide the proctor with knowledge of their learner's baseline skill level and motivation
Nonmalleable curriculum	• Set curriculum that does not respond to trainee needs or changes in policy and technology • Course content should be revised regularly (eg, every 6 mo)
No learner assessment	• Precourse and postcourse assessment provides objective evidence of learning and course validity
Lack of content regarding common pitfalls	• "Expert tips" participants are looking for often are how to get out of trouble, and how to anticipate hurdles and common pitfalls • Create ways to practice dealing with these pitfalls, and providing didactic teaching
Lack of inclusion of team building and stakeholder relations skills	• One of the most difficult pieces of introducing a new MIS technique is achieving stakeholder buy-in and creating a viable, working team around the surgeon • Courses should include these important nontechnical skills
Lack of follow-up	• Ongoing mentorship in one form or another is necessary for improved implantation of skills once trainee returns to home site (eg, video review, submission of outcomes, ongoing communication with staff running course)

quality of videos and most often use society Web sites requiring membership login. Sources most accessed include YouTube, SCORE portal, ORLive, Access Surgery, and Websurg.[39,40]

However, this newly available resource, holding educational promise, has questionable quality control.[41] In a study of available laparoscopic colectomy videos online, Celentano and colleagues[42] found, not surprisingly, only 18.6% of laparoscopic right hemicolectomy videos underwent peer-review process before publication. There is some danger in open access availability of training resources if they demonstrate inadequate, unsafe technique. This was illustrated by Deal and Alseidi[43] who show a failure to achieve of a critical view of safety by the most operating surgeons in laparoscopic cholecystectomy videos online (1 of 160 videos). Video-review as a training resource in the MIS training armamentarium is already occurring, and it is the responsibility of MIS trainers worldwide to create a reliable, regulated, and open-access resource of high-quality surgical video.

MENTORING AND COACHING

Despite the burgeoning number of MIS fellowship programs, there are still limited continuing professional development opportunities for mature surgeons hoping to develop MIS skills. A positive trend for staff surgeons is incorporating peer mentoring or coaching (proctorship) into their practice.[44] Mentors can be peers, or senior surgeons, who have more advanced skills and are willing to share their knowledge with others. Numerous creative mentoring platforms exist, including electronic platforms (as simple as a closed group in Facebook) in which less experienced surgeons share videos and ideas, looking for input. With the first generation of MIS surgeons now getting toward retirement, there is full complement of would-be mentors to stand beside new trainees. Miskovic and colleagues[45] have shown the positive outcomes of mentoring for advanced laparoscopic colorectal cases. Significantly higher rates of conversion have been noted in nonmentored laparoscopic colorectal cases of surgeons who took a short course only, compared with those in which the surgeon new to the technique is being mentored.

Coaching is subtly different. Similar to professional athletics, a coach does not actually have to be personally excellent at the activity. A coach's goal, after discussing the trainee's objectives, is to observe performance one-on-one and make observations for improvement. It is less about, "hey, be more like me,", and more about, "how you can be better."[46]

Gawande[47] helped popularize the idea of professional coaching. If top professional athletes and successful musicians pay coaches to encourage their continued improvement and excellence, why can't surgeons? "The coach provides the outside eyes and ears, and makes you aware of where you're falling short. This is tricky. Human beings resist exposure and critique; our brains are well defended. So coaches use a variety of approaches—showing what other, respected colleagues do, for instance, or reviewing videos of the subject's performance. The most common, however, is just conversation."[47]

Qualities of a successful peer-coaching session in the OR include a relationship of collaboration, self-evaluation of areas for improvement by the trainee, and honest feedback provided by the coach with a focus on amplification of capacity.[48,49] Palter and colleagues[35] performed an RCT to contrast mature surgeons advancing their laparoscopic suturing skills with a peer-coaching program compared with a conventional didactic course. Surgeons who participated in the coaching arm showed significantly improved skill acquisition. This is a key moment-in-time to consider incorporating coaching into MIS oncology training and address the limitations of the current continuing professional development model.

A FEW SOUND EDUCATIONAL PRINCIPLES
Curriculum Development

A complete discussion of curricular design is well beyond the scope of this review. However, for any surgeon interested in MIS training curriculum or program design, a six-step approach, modeled briefly in **Fig. 1**, is suggested by Thomas and co-workers.[50] Their model highlights three common pitfalls in educational programs.

The first is that most teachers fail to take a moment to ask, "What do learners know already, and what don't they know?". Often experts sit in a dark room and decide the goals and objectives of a learning program. A true needs assessment occurs in concert with the learners.

A second pitfall is a mismatch between the goals and objectives of a curriculum and the strategy that is used to accomplish them. For example, if laparoscopic hemorrhage control is recognized as an issue, a lecture is unlikely to be the most effective way to combat the problem. Unfortunately, this happens all the time. The simplest strategy is often not the best or most educationally effective.

Along a similar line, the third common curriculum design pitfall is using assessment methods that are completely inappropriate for what is being assessed. If a trainer is hoping to assess whether his or her trainee can demonstrate proficiency in intracorporeal suturing, an multiple choice question (MCQ) examination or inanimate model does not provide the needed assessment information. A more appropriate assessment device is actually observing the trainee's intraoperative performance.

Learning Curves

It is widely accepted that the adoption of a new technique requires an implementation period during which learning occurs and outcomes may not be as good. This time

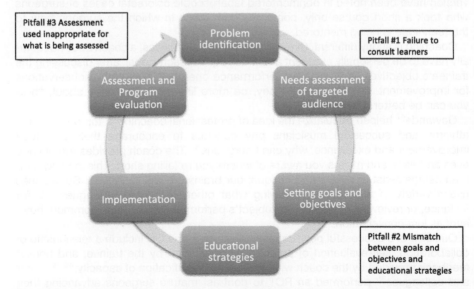

Fig. 1. Six-step approach to minimally invasive surgery. (*Data from* Thomas P, Kern D, Hughes M, et al. Six-step approach to curriculum development in medical education. Boston: Johns Hopkins University Press; 2016.)

period is called the learning curve. Methods to reduce the slope and speed up time to plateau of MIS learning curves occupy significant space in the MIS training literature, including using new technology and simulation to facilitate.[51] Colorectal surgeons have done a lot of work in this area and since the 1990s have been tracking outcomes to identify learning curves for laparoscopic right and left hemicolectomy.[52,53] SAGES has confirmed that performing 20 procedures is necessary to attain the level of expertise required for curative oncologic surgery in laparoscopic colon cancer, based on results of the COST trial.[54] It is important to understand that these are not steadfast numbers, and learning curves have the capacity to be shortened. Conversely, surgical volume does not necessarily translate into quality and patient safety. Transfer of knowledge, proctorship, and breaking down advanced procedures into discrete principles and tasks can shorten learning curves drastically.[55,56]

Assessment and Feedback

An essential tenet of educational theory ensures that students receive assessment based on predefined learning objectives in a formative (feedback) and summative (final assessment) fashion.[9] There are many examples of validated assessment tools (eg, GOALS[57] and MISTELS[58] for laparoscopic skills, and GEARS[59] for robotic skills) that are available for immediate use in MIS training programs. Most of these tools assess basic MIS skills or procedures, such as cholecystectomy.[60] Although originally developed for use in the simulated environment, these tools have the capacity to enhance perioperative feedback that has been shown to optimally stimulate learning and skill acquisition.[61] Providing focused feedback as soon after performance as possible is essential for learning motor skills given that trainee analysis and processing are linked to the perceived tactile information received during the procedure.[1]

Program Examples

There is notable variety in quality and organization of MIS training programs. Here we describe the implementation of a national Laparoscopic Colorectal Surgery training program in England and the evolution of a standardized robotics training program that show strong curricular design elements.

National Training Program for Laparoscopic Colorectal Surgery

Laparoscopic colorectal surgeons in England in the early 2000s had unacceptably high complication and conversion rates. At this time, only 5% of general surgeons performing LCS were trained to perform it, even though it was a national standard to offer this surgery. Given the long learning curve, and evidence showing that surgeons without fellowship training had worse outcomes, the Imperial College of London began the National Training Programme for Laparoscopic Colorectal Surgery in 2008.[62–64] The goal was to create confident laparoscopic colorectal surgeons through national distribution of expertise.

As seen in **Fig. 2**, trainees in the program follow a strict advancement algorithm as they progress toward independence. Each step is monitored by a proctor, and documented. An objective, validated assessment tool (Competency Assessment Tool) has been developed ensure surgeons are ready to independently and safely perform laparoscopic colon surgery (**Fig. 3**).[65] The Competency Assessment Tool was validated in the OR as a workplace-based assessment tool and comes with a written report card of feedback. This feedback directs failing candidates on how to improve and also helps passing candidates continue to move toward mastery. All candidates involved in its validation were surgeons certified by the

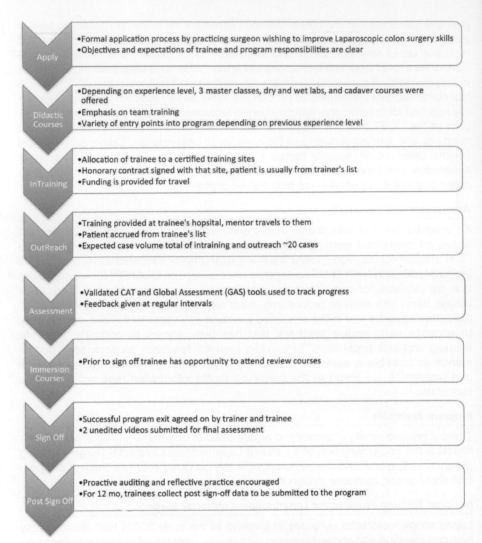

Apply
- Formal application process by practicing surgeon wishing to improve Laparoscopic colon surgery skills
- Objectives and expectations of trainee and program responsibilities are clear

Didactic Courses
- Depending on experience level, 3 master classes, dry and wet labs, and cadaver courses were offered
- Emphasis on team training
- Variety of entry points into program depending on previous experience level

InTraining
- Allocation of trainee to a certified training sites
- Honorary contract signed with that site, patient is usually from trainer's list
- Funding is provided for travel

OutReach
- Training provided at trainee's hopsital, mentor travels to them
- Patient accrued from trainee's list
- Expected case volume total of intraining and outreach ~20 cases

Assessment
- Validated CAT and Global Assessment (GAS) tools used to track progress
- Feedback given at regular intervals

Immersion Courses
- Prior to sign off trainee has opportunity to attend review courses

Sign Off
- Successful program exit agreed on by trainer and trainee
- 2 unedited videos submitted for final assessment

Post Sign Off
- Proactive auditing and reflective practice encouraged
- For 12 mo, trainees collect post sign-off data to be submitted to the program

Fig. 2. Structure of National Training Program for laparoscopic colorectal surgery in England. CAT, Competency Assessment Tool. (*Data from* About the programme. Lapco National Training Programme for laparoscopic colorectal surgery. 2015. Available at: http://lapco.nhs.uk/. Accessed December 20, 2017)

Imperial College of London and deemed to be competent to run an independent general surgery practice. Arguably the greatest success of this national program is the level of program evaluation and study that was built into the process. Participants were required to track their outcomes, continuing for 1 year after involvement in the program.

Overall, the laparoscopic colorectal program has been successful. In 2011, Coleman and colleagues[62] reported that the proportion of colorectal surgery performed laparoscopically had risen from 13.8% in 2007 to 33% in 2010 (one of the highest provision rates of LCS in Europe). Surgical outcomes for the first 816 cases showed performance levels equivalent to expert surgeon's data, including hospital stay (5 days),

LAPAROSCOPIC COLORECTAL RESECTION

Trainee ID [ ] Assessor ID [ ] Case No. [ ] Date [ ]   © 2010 Imperial College London

TASK	INSTRUMENTATION	SKILLS	ERRORS	END-PRODUCT
EXPOSURE — Port insertion/ placement:		**Manipulating small bowel:**	**This task was performed with:**	**Was the operating field sufficiently exposed?**
Hazardous	Dangerous insertion or wrong position	Hazardous — Uncontrolled movements, insufficient view	Perforation/ bleeding — Macroscopic perforation, burn or grasp marks, bleed	No — Anatomical landmarks not properly identified
Imprecise	Incomplete insertion or ergonomically poor position	Laborious — Awkward and repeated attempts, ineffective	Near miss — Bloody dissection, too close to sensitive structures	Vaguely — Main structures identified but incomplete exposure
Safe	Safe insertion and ergonomically good position	Effective — Meaningful adjustment of NDH to improve exposure	No damage — No damage to bowel, major blood vessels	Yes — Main structures identified and exposed
Versatile	Masterful insertion, ideal positioning	Expeditious — Strategic and intelligent adjustments by NDH	Tissue-protective — Performed with best possible tissue protection	Anatomically — Crystal clear demonstration of anatomy
N/A		N/A	N/A	N/A
PEDICLE CONTROL — Use of haemostatic tool (clip applier/ diathermy/ stapler):		**Dissection of vessels:**	**This task was performed with:**	**How was the management of the vascular pedicle?**
Hazardous	Insufficient view, uncontrolled movements	Hazardous — Insufficient view, uncontrolled movements	Perforation/ bleeding — Macroscopic perforation, burn or grasp marks, bleed	Uncontrolled — Haemostasis unsafe, grossly at wrong level
Laborious	Awkward and repeated unnecessary attempts	Inefficient — Several, hesitant cuts	Near miss — Bloody dissection, too close to sensitive structures	Imprecise — Safe but inefficient, non-ideal level
Efficient	Instrument accurately placed and engaged	Safe — Safe dissection under view	No damage — No damage to bowel, major blood vessels	Safe — Vessels safely secured, correct level
Masterly	Highly efficient and safe use of instrument	Efficient — Smooth and efficient dissection	Tissue-protective — Performed with best possible tissue protection	Flawless — Vessels efficiently secured, ideal level
N/A		N/A	N/A	N/A
MOBILISATION — Use of graspers/ dissection tools:		**Anatomical dissection technique:**	**This task was performed with:**	**Was the large bowel safely mobilised and were the landmarks identified?**
Uncoordinated	Stiff and uncontrolled movements, overshooting	Flawed — Wrong tissue plane, unable to correct quickly	Perforation/ bleeding — Macroscopic perforation, burn or grasp marks, bleed	No — Inadequate mobilisation, landmarks not identified
Hesitant	Controlled movements, but hesitant and inefficient	Imprecise — Repeatedly wrong tissue plane, able to correct	Near miss — Bloody dissection, too close to sensitive structures	Insufficiently — Partial mobilisation, landmarks defined
Skilful	Smooth, controlled and meaningful movements	Safe — Rarely wrong plane, able to correct quickly	No damage — No damage to bowel, major blood vessels	Yes — Sufficient mobilisation, landmarks defined
Versatile	Masterful instrument use, effective movements	Meticulous — Constantly stays in correct tissue plane	Tissue-protective — Performed with best possible tissue protection	Ideal — Flawless mobilisation, perfect landmark definition
N/A		N/A	N/A	N/A
RESECTION — Use of intestinal stapler:		**Preparation of large bowel for resection:**	**This task was performed with:**	**How was the resection and anastomosis performed?**
Hazardous	Stiff and uncontrolled movements, overshooting	Hazardous — Insufficient views, uncontrolled movements	Perforation/ bleeding — Macroscopic perforation, burn or grasp marks, bleed	Faulty — Likely to compromise integrity of anastomosis
Laborious	Awkward and repeated unnecessary attempts	Inefficient — Hesitant and awkward dissection technique	Near miss — Bloody dissection, too close to sensitive structures	Suboptimal — Stump management, safe anastomosis
Efficient	Instrument accurately placed and engaged	Safe — Safe dissection under view	No damage — No damage to bowel, major blood vessels	Safe — Adequate resection level, safe anastomosis
Masterly	Highly efficient and safe use of instrument	Efficient — Smooth and efficient dissection technique	Tissue-protective — Performed with best possible tissue protection	Ideal — Ideal stump management, perfect anastomosis
N/A		N/A	N/A	N/A

Fig. 3. The Competency Assessment Tool for laparoscopic colorectal surgery. (*From* Miskovic D, Ni M, Wyles S, et al. Is competency assessment at the specialist level achievable? A study for the National Training Programme in laparoscopic colorectal surgery in England. Ann Surg 2013;257:479; with permission.)

reoperation rate (3.6%), leak rate (2.6%), in-hospital mortality (0.5%), and total complication rate (14.3%). These equivalent outcome data were sustained in the year following trainee sign-off. Overall, the program offers a replicable archetype for advanced MIS training of other oncologic procedures.

Developing a Robotics Curriculum

Implementation of robotic surgery has increased exponentially in the last decade. In Europe, urologists use robotic techniques most often, whereas in North America, it is gynecologists and general surgeons who are leading the field.[59,66] The skills required for competence in robotic surgery unique from laparoscopic surgery include use of the console and docking, greater degrees of freedom with a variety of different instruments, and lack of haptic feedback. Seeing the results of movements on different tissue types, in a variety of patients, takes practice and continued self-evaluation for the surgeon. It has been shown that surgeons who have laparoscopic skills develop robotic skills at a quicker pace,[67,68] and therefore specialists require less training hours than those starting from scratch.[69]

Similar to the early days of laparoscopic surgery, extent of training before performing robotic procedures varies widely and concerns for patient safety (because of lack of formal certification programs) has developed. In search of a roadmap for overcoming the steep robotics learning curve, Sridhar and colleagues[59] developed a curricular framework that exhibits strong educational principles (**Fig. 4**). This curriculum is based on a visioning process of international experts[69] and their experience with a fellowship program.[59] Technical skill objectives are divided into two categories: patient-side (eg, docking, establishing pneumoperitoneum) and console-based skills. Their curriculum emphasizes modular environments beginning in the classroom,

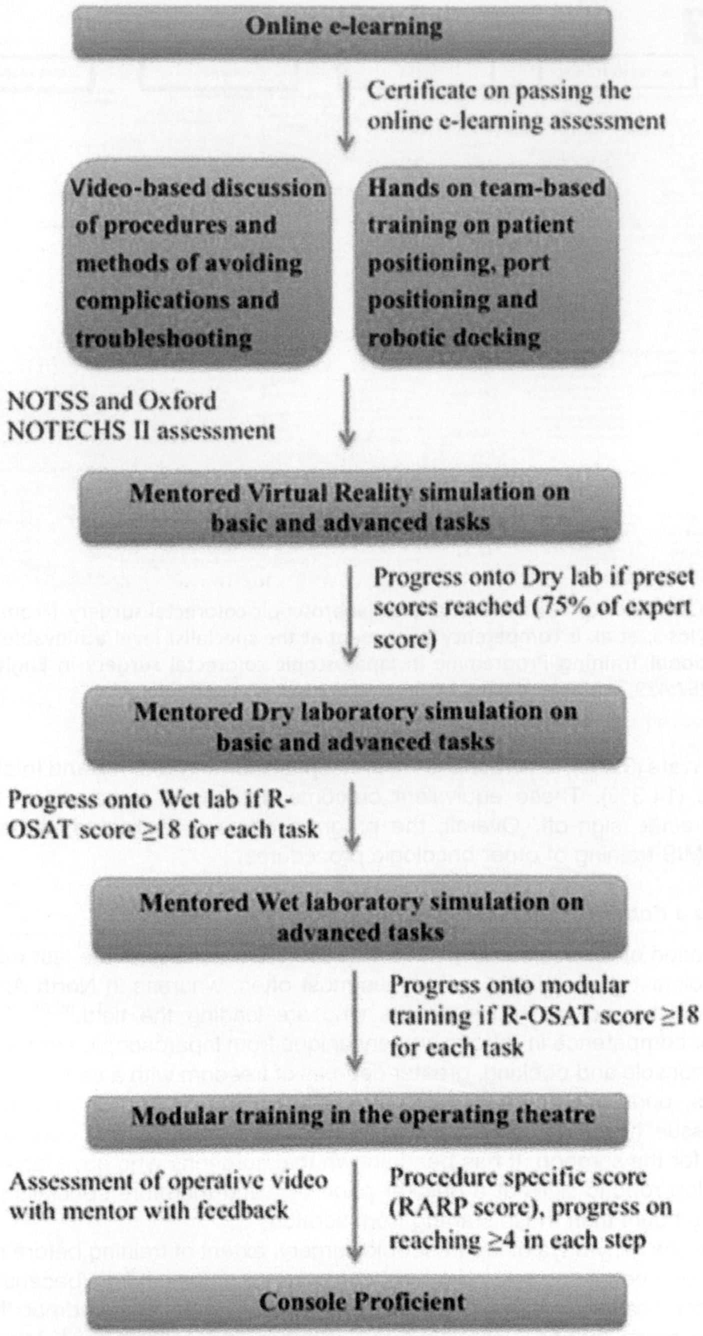

Online e-learning

Certificate on passing the
online e-learning assessment

Video-based discussion of procedures and methods of avoiding complications and troubleshooting

Hands on team-based training on patient positioning, port positioning and robotic docking

NOTSS and Oxford
NOTECHS II assessment

Mentored Virtual Reality simulation on basic and advanced tasks

Progress onto Dry lab if preset
scores reached (75% of expert
score)

Mentored Dry laboratory simulation on basic and advanced tasks

Progress onto Wet lab if R-
OSAT score ≥18 for each task

Mentored Wet laboratory simulation on advanced tasks

Progress onto modular
training if R-OSAT score ≥18
for each task

Modular training in the operating theatre

Assessment of operative video
with mentor with feedback

Procedure specific score
(RARP score), progress on
reaching ≥4 in each step

Console Proficient

Fig. 4. Proposed curricular model for training in robotic surgery. (*From* Sridhar A, Briggs T, Kelly J, et al. Training in robotic surgery: an overview. Curr Urol Rep 2017;18:58; with permission.)

relocating to the simulation laboratory and to a virtual console, and finally to the OR. A natural regression of responsibility of the trainer occurs throughout the process. They begin as a preceptor, stepping in to correct often and eventually transition into a proctor, supervising only and allowing trainee independence. Within each environment there are processes that begin with the trainee performing the simplest part of the procedure and progressively assuming responsibility for more complex portions of the operation.

Dual console technology is an interesting addition to the training repertoire for robotic surgery.[70] Both the surgeon and the trainee have access to the patient with their own console. Although associated with a substantial increase in cost, trainers are able to step in and take over immediately without the trainee having to leave the console or even switch places. Smith and colleagues[71] showed that this provided the trainee with more operating time on the console but did not increase overall operative length or change outcomes.

Continual research is needed to support the hypothesis that robotic MIS produces similar oncologic outcomes at all levels of training, given that current research supports only feasibility data at large.

Nontechnical Skills and Team-Based Training

Sridhar and coworkers[59] robotics curriculum includes nontechnical and team-based training. In open surgery, nearly 90% of intraoperative errors were systems errors and 40% were related to failures in team communication.[72,73] With the complexity of the robotic system, it is not hard to imagine that precise communication is even more crucial.[59] Nontechnical skills, such as a teamwork, leadership, decision-making, and situational awareness, are teachable and have been shown to have significant impact on surgical outcomes.[74] A recent systematic review by Wood and colleagues[75] looked at nontechnical skill assessment for surgeons and recommended the NOTSS (Nontechnical Skills for Surgeons) as the gold standard tool for individual training, and the NOTECHS for team-based training.

Impact of Minimally Invasive Surgery Training on Resident Training

A key, albeit controversial, discussion relating to robotics is how this new technology has affected resident operative time. Generally, as robotic-assisted cases are introduced into general surgical programs a concomitant decrease in laparoscopic cases occurs.[76] This has caused an upward shift in level of trainee operating and major reduction in resident time operating. The MIS revolution has occurred concurrently with increasing numbers of fellows in the OR and decreased resident duty hours. Resident operating time, it can be argued, is at an all-time low.[66,77]

EXCITING NEW DEVELOPMENTS
Patient-Specific Virtual Reality Simulation Modeling

Professional racers take time to run a new course before competing; actors ensure they have a dress rehearsal. Should surgeons rehearse a high-intensity case? Patient-specific VR (PSVR) is the next generation of how VR-simulators can be used for more than generic skill practice. PSVR uses a patient's preoperative imaging to create a VR model specific to their case, including specific vascular and anatomic details. Both the preprocedural planning (cognitive) and the physical movement (psychomotor) rehearsal benefits have been well documented in other fields, such as aerospace engineering and in the military.[78] PSVR is currently used most often in endovascular surgery,[79] and Suzuki and colleagues[80] in Japan have created a

PSVR model for laparoscopic colectomy. Whole team rehearsal of a particularly difficult case has also been performed.[81]

To be able to predictably rehearse the complex portions of an elective operation before proceeding with the real-life patient's case holds promise for patient safety and surgical outcomes. It is well known that anatomic bench models have a training ceiling beyond which a trainee receives limited benefit by practicing on them. This may be one answer to raising the simulation ceiling.[15] Although still in the prototype phase, PSVR has the potential to create simulated full-procedure exercises with high fidelity.

Game-Based Training

Knowledge and skills acquired during game play have been shown to translate to performance of real world tasks and draw on the motivational goals of competition. Skills exhibited by experienced video gamers are largely similar to those acquired by MIS surgeons (eg, hand-eye coordination, high level of concentration on tasks).[82] In 2016, a systematic review of five RCTs looked for a correlation between video games and laparoscopic performance. Two of the studies showed a reduction in error after the use of video games and one showed an increased speed of task completion for three of four laparoscopic tasks after preparation using video games. To date there has been no study of how video game learning translates to laparoscopic skill in the OR.[83]

On a similar note, El Beheiry and colleagues[84] demonstrated that adding an element of serious game competition into a standard simulation curriculum at the residency level stimulated skill development and time to completion of the course. Despite good evidence that simulator use increases laparoscopic skill, getting trainees to use available skill centers (even those with after-hours access) remains a challenge experienced far and wide by program directors.[85] Serious games, mental contests with a primarily educational goal, address the motivational challenge and provide external motivation for trainees.[86] The serious game skills competition involved in the study by El Beheiry and coworkers[84] was simple, involving six fundamental skill challenges on a VR simulator. Many other platforms are already in development, including some showing improved technical skills during robotics training[87] and a simulator helping trainees recognize and troubleshoot equipment-related MIS problems that would occur in the OR (**Fig. 5**).[88] Incorporating video game–style VR simulators and serious game skill competitions into training programs could break up the monotony of repetitive practice.[89]

Telementoring

Telementoring is an evolving technology that allows an expert mentor to observe and provide advice without being in the room (synchronous and asynchronous). SAGES defines telementoring as, "a relationship, facilitated by telecommunication technology, in which an expert (mentor) provided guidance to a less experienced learner (mentee) from a remote location."[33] In its most basic form, intraoperative video is broadcast to the mentor's office, and in this way, the observing surgeon can interact in real time with the operating surgeon. This interaction occurs either by verbal instruction or, in some cases, visually through a pointer tool on the screen (**Fig. 6**).

In robotics, telementoring has been taken a step further. The surgical mentor can now "extend their hands into the remote operating room," controlling the instruments from afar and participating in the surgery physically.[90] This is termed teleassisting. Telementoring is emerging as a cost-effective and practical alternative proctoring tool that prevents mentors from having to travel excessively and take time off from work.[91]

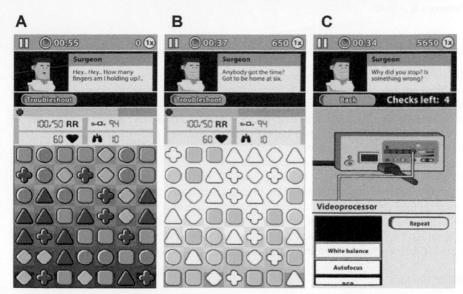

Fig. 5. Graafland and colleagues' serious game. (*A*) Main screen, with mini-game (*bottom*), the patient's vital signs, and a supervising surgeon (*above*). (*B*) During the mini-game, the player deals with problem scenarios that resemble real-life problems in MIS, such as the blurred screen. (*C*) After the player recognizes the problem scenario, he or she can solve it by selecting the correct action on a simulation of the MIS equipment. (*From* Graafland M, Bemelman W, Schijven M. Game-based training improves the surgeon's situational awareness in the operation room: a randomized controlled trial. Surg Endosc 2017;31:4095; with permission.)

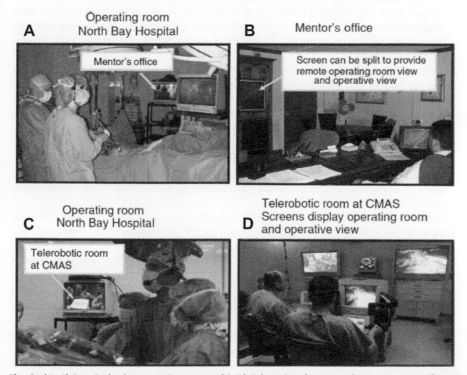

Fig. 6. (*A, B*) Surgical telementoring setup. (*C, D*) Teleassisted surgery. (*From* Hung A, Chen J, Shah A, et al. Telementoring and telesurgery for minimally invasive procedures. J Urol 2018;199:6; with permission.)

SUMMARY

There are a wide variety of available training opportunities for residents, fellows, and surgical oncologists looking to advance their MIS oncology skills. These range from take-home tablet bench models to fellowships and international mentoring opportunities, to lifelike simulations that allow realistic simulated practice sessions of advanced procedures. Despite an incredible growth of technological development, the range of quality and organization of MIS training programs has never been so variable or ad hoc. Here we have introduced a common standard to strive for, with examples of programs that are working hard to promote educational and oncologic excellence. Technology is advancing in leaps and bounds, and its potential for incorporation into advanced MIS training is stunning. The new training opportunities found in exciting advances, such as telementoring, serious game technology, and thoughtful instruction by mentors who now have more than 30 years of MIS oncology experience make it exciting to observe the progress of the next 30 years.

REFERENCES

1. Poulin E, Gagne J, Boushey R. Advanced laparoscopic skills acquisition: the case of laparoscopic colorectal surgery. Surg Clin North Am 2006;86:987–1004.
2. Society of American Gastrointestinal and Endoscopic Surgeons (SAGES). Integrating advanced laparoscopy into surgical residency training: a SAGES Position Paper. 2009. Available at: https://www.sages.org/publications/guidelines/integrating-advanced-laparoscopy-into-surgical-residency-training-a-sages-position-paper/. Accessed December 20, 2017.
3. Richards M, McAteer J, Drake T, et al. A national review of the frequency of minimally invasive surgery among general surgery residents assessment of ACGME case logs during 2 decades of general surgery resident training. JAMA Surg 2015;150(2):169–72.
4. Rosser J, Murayama M, Gabriel N. Minimally invasive surgical training solutions for the twenty-first century. Surg Clin North Am 2000;80(5):1607–24.
5. Wakabayashi G, Cherqui D, Geller D, et al. Recommendations for laparoscopic liver resection: a report from the second international consensus conference held in Morioka. Ann Surg 2015;261(4):619–29.
6. Buell J, Thomas M, Rudich S, et al. Experience with more than 500 minimally invasive hepatic procedures. Ann Surg 2008;248:475–86.
7. Imura S, Shimada M, Utsunomiya T, et al. Current status of laparoscopic liver surgery in Japan: results of a multicenter Japanese experience. Surg Today 2014; 44:1214–9.
8. Yamada S, Shimada M, Imura S, et al. Effective stepwise training and procedure standardization for young surgeons to perform laparoscopic left hepatectomy. Surg Endosc 2017;31:2623–9.
9. Fried G, Feldman L, Vassiliou M, et al. Proving the value of simulation in laparoscopic surgery. Ann Surg 2004;240:518–28.
10. Gurusamy K, Aggarwal R, Palanivelu L, et al. Systematic review of randomized controlled trials on the effectiveness of virtual reality training for laparoscopic surgery. Br J Surg 2008;95:1088–97.
11. Nagendran M, Gurusamy KS, Aggarwal R, et al. Virtual reality training for surgical trainees in laparoscopic surgery. Cochrane Database Syst Rev 2009;8(1): CD006575.
12. Grantcharov T, Kristiansen V, Bendix J, et al. Randomized clinical trial of virtual reality simulation for laparoscopic skills training. Br J Surg 2004;91:146–50.

13. Moulton C, Dubrowski A, Macrae H, et al. Teaching surgical skills: what kind of practice makes perfect? A randomized controlled trial. Ann Surg 2006;244: 400–9.
14. Thinggaard E, Kleif J, Bjerrum F. Off-site training of laparoscopic skills, a scoping review using a thematic analysis. Surg Endosc 2016;30:4733–41.
15. Beyer-Berjot L, Palter V, Grantcharov T, et al. Advanced training in laparoscopic abdominal surgery: a systematic review. Surgery 2014;156:676–88.
16. Reznick R, MacRae H. Teaching surgical skills-changes in the wind. N Engl J Med 2006;355:2664–9.
17. Essani R, Scriven R, McLarty A. Simulated laparoscopic sigmoidectomy training: responsiveness of surgery residents. Dis Colon Rectum 2009;52:1956–61.
18. Palter VN, Grantcharov TP. Development and validation of a comprehensive curriculum to teach an advanced minimally invasive procedure: a randomized controlled trial. Ann Surg 2012;256:25–32.
19. Zevin B, Levy JS, Satava RM, et al. A consensus based framework for design, validation, and implementation of simulation-based training curricula in surgery. J Am Coll Surg 2012;215:580–6.e3.
20. Gala R, Orejuela F, Gerten K, et al. Effect of validated skills simulation on operating room performance in obstetrics and gynecology residents. Obstet Gynecol 2013;121:578–84.
21. Aggarwal R, Ward J, Balasundaram I, et al. Proving the effectiveness of virtual reality simulation for training in laparoscopic surgery. Ann Surg 2007;246:771–9.
22. Ramos P, Montez J, Tripp A, et al. Face, content, construct and concurrent validity of dry laboratory exercises for robotic training using a global assessment tool. BJU Int 2014;113(5):836–42.
23. Hung A, Jayaratna I, Teruya K, et al. Comparative assessment of three standardized robotic surgery training methods. BJU Int 2013;112(6):864–71.
24. Park A, Kavic S, Lee T, et al. Minimally invasive surgery: the evolution of fellowship. Surgery 2007;142:505–13.
25. Fellowship Council. Statement of past chairman. Available at: https://fellowshipcouncil.org/about/. Accessed December 21, 2017.
26. Bell R, Banker M, Rhodes R, et al. Graduate medical education in surgery in the United States. Surg Clin North Am 2007;87(4):811–23.
27. Numann P. Presidential Address American College of Surgeons: stewardship of our profession. Bull Am Coll Surg 2011;(Dec):24–8.
28. Jokinen E, Mikkola T, Harkki P. Evaluation of a web course on the basics of gynecological laparoscopy in resident training. J Surg Educ 2017;74:717–23.
29. Ellaway R, Masters K. AMEE guide 32: e-learning in medical education. Part 1: learning, teaching and assessment. Med Teach 2008;30(5):455–73.
30. Jayakumar N, Brunckhorst O, Dasgupta P, et al. e-Learning in surgical education: a systematic review. J Surg Educ 2015;72(6):1145–57.
31. de Rooij T, van Hilst J, Boerma D, et al. Impact of a nationwide training program in minimally invasive distal pancreatectomy (LAELAPS). Ann Surg 2016;264(5): 754–62.
32. Heniford B, Backus C, Matthews B, et al. Optimal teaching environment for laparoscopic splenectomy. Am J Surg 2001;181:226–30.
33. Schlachta C, Nguyen N, Ponsky T, et al. Project 6 Summit: SAGES telementoring initiative. Surg Endosc 2016;30:3665–72.
34. Cuesta M, van der Wielen N, Straatman J, et al. Mastering minimally invasive esophagectomy requires a mentor; experience of a personal mentorship. Ann Med Surg (Lond) 2017;13:38–41.

35. Palter V, Beyfuss K, Jokhio A, et al. Peer coaching to teach faculty surgeons an advanced laparoscopic skill: a randomized controlled trial. Surgery 2016;160: 1392–9.
36. Shea C, Wright D, Whiteacre C. Actual and observational practice: unique perspective on learning. Res Q Exerc Sport 1993;67(March Suppl):A–79.
37. Crawshaw B, Steele S, Lee E, et al. Failing to prepare is preparing to fail: a single-blinded, randomized controlled trial to determine the impact of a preoperative instructional video on the ability of residents to perform laparoscopic right colectomy. Dis Colon Rectum 2016;59:28–34.
38. Mota P, Carvalho N, Carvalho-Dias E, et al. Video-based surgical learning: improving trainee education and preparation for surgery. J Surg Educ 2018; 75(3):828–35.
39. Rapp A, Healy M, Charlton M, et al. YouTube is the most frequently used educational video source for surgical preparation. J Surg Educ 2016;73(6):1072–6.
40. Pape-Koehler C, Immenroth M, Sauerland S, et al. Multimedia-based training on Internet platforms improves surgical performance: a randomized controlled trial. Surg Endosc 2013;27(5):1737–47.
41. Frongia G, Mehrabi A, Fonouni H, et al. YouTube as a potential training resource for laparoscopic fundoplication. J Surg Educ 2016;73:1066–71.
42. Celentano V, Browning M, Hitchins C, et al. Training value of laparoscopic colorectal videos on the World Wide Web: a pilot study on the educational quality of laparoscopic right hemicolectomy videos. Surg Endosc 2017;31:4496–504.
43. Deal S, Alseidi A. Concerns of quality and safety in public domain surgical education videos: an assessment of the critical view of safety in frequently used laparoscopic cholecystectomy videos. J Am Coll Surg 2017;225:725–30.
44. Bonrath E, Dedy N, Gordon L, et al. Comprehensive surgical coaching enhances surgical skill in the operating room. Ann Surg 2015;262:205–12.
45. Miskovic D, Wyles S, Ni M, et al. Systematic review on mentoring and simulation in laparoscopic colorectal surgery. Ann Surg 2010;252:943–51.
46. Mutabdzic D, Mylopoulos M, Murnaghan M, et al. Coaching surgeons. Ann Surg 2015;262:213–6.
47. Gawande A. Personal best: top athletes and singers have coaches. Should you? In: New Yorker magazine. 2011. Available at: https://www.newyorker.com/magazine/2011/10/03/personal-best. Accessed December 15, 2017.
48. Schwellnus H, Carnahan H. Peer coaching with health care professionals: what is the current status of the literature and what are the key components necessary in peercoaching? A scoping review. Med Teach 2014;36:38–46.
49. Greenberg C, Ghousseini H, Pavuluri Quamme S, et al. Surgical coaching for individual performance improvement. Ann Surg 2015;261:32–4.
50. Thomas P, Kern D, Hughes M, et al. Curriculum development for medical education: a six-step approach. Boston: Johns Hopkins University Press; 2016.
51. Kowalewski K, Hendrie J, Schmidt M, et al. Validation of the mobile serious game application Touch Surgery™ for cognitive training and assessment of laparoscopic cholecystectomy. Surg Endosc 2017;31:4058–66.
52. Schlachta C, Mamazza J, Seshadri P, et al. Defining a learning curve for laparoscopic colorectal resections. Dis Colon Rectum 2001;44:217–22.
53. Dincler S, Koller MT, Steurer J, et al. Multidimensional analysis of learning curves in laparoscopic sigmoid resection: eight-year results. Dis Colon Rectum 2003;46: 1371–8.

54. Clinical Outcomes of Surgical Therapy Study Group (COST). A comparison of laparoscopically assisted and open colectomy for colon cancer. N Engl J Med 2004;350(20):2050–9.
55. Ericsson K. Acquisition and maintenance of medical expertise: a perspective from the expert-performance approach with deliberate practice. Acad Med 2015;90:1471–86.
56. Hashimoto D, Sirimanna P, Gomez E, et al. Deliberate practice enhances quality of laparoscopic surgical performance in a randomized controlled trial: from arrested development to expert performance. Surg Endosc 2015;29: 3154–62.
57. Scott D, Bergen P, Rege R, et al. Laparoscopic training on bench models: better and more cost effective than operating room experience? J Am Coll Surg 2000; 191:272–83.
58. Vassiliou M, Ghitulescu G, Feldman L, et al. The MISTELS program to measure technical skill in laparoscopic surgery: evidence for reliability. Surg Endosc 2006;20:744–7.
59. Sridhar A, Briggs T, Kelly J, et al. Training in robotic surgery: an overview. Curr Urol Rep 2017;18:58.
60. Watanabe U, Bilgic E, Lebedeva, et al. A systematic review of performance assessment tools for laparoscopic cholecystectomy. Surg Endosc 2016;30: 832–44.
61. McKendy K, Watanabe Y, Lee L, et al. Perioperative feedback in surgical training: a systematic review. Am J Surg 2017;214:117–26.
62. Coleman M, Hanna G, Kennedy R. The National Training Programme for laparoscopic colorectal surgery in England: a new training paradigm. Colorectal Dis 2011;13:614–6.
63. Tekkis P, Senagore A, Delaney C, et al. Evaluation of the learning curve in laparoscopic colorectal surgery: comparison of right-sided and left-sided resections. Ann Surg 2005;242:83–91.
64. Kirchhoff P, Dincler S, Buchmann P. A multivariate analysis of potential risk factors for intra- and postoperative complications in 1316 elective laparoscopic colorectal procedures. Ann Surg 2008;248:259–65.
65. Miskovic D, Ni M, Wyles S, et al. Is competency assessment at the specialist level achievable? A study for the National Training Programme in laparoscopic colorectal surgery in England. Ann Surg 2013;257:476–82.
66. Mehaffey J, Michaels A, Mullen M, et al. Adoption of robotics in a general surgery residency program: at what cost? J Surg Res 2017;213:269–73.
67. Angell J, Gomez MS, Baig MM, et al. Contribution of laparoscopic training to robotic proficiency. J Endourol 2013;27(8):1027–31.
68. Kilic GS, Walsh TM, Borahay M, et al. Effect of residents' previous laparoscopic surgery experience on initial robotic suturing experience. ISRN Obstet Gynecol 2012;2012:569456.
69. Ahmed K, Khan R, Mottrie A, et al. Development of a standardised training curriculum for robotic surgery: a consensus statement from an international multidisciplinary group of experts. BJU Int 2015,116(1):93–101.
70. Foote J, Valea F. Robotic surgical training: where are we? Gynecol Oncol 2016; 143:179–83.
71. Smith A, Scott E, Krivak T, et al. Dual-console robotic surgery: a new teaching paradigm. J Robot Surg 2013;7(2):113–8.
72. Gawande A, Zinner M, Studdert D, et al. Analysis of errors reported by surgeons at three teaching hospitals. Surgery 2003;133(6):614–21.

73. Bogner M. Misadventures in health care. Mahwah (NJ): Psychology Press; 2008.
74. Yule S, Flin R, Paterson-Brown S, et al. Non-technical skills for surgeons in the operating room: a review of the literature. Surgery 2006;139(2):140–9.
75. Wood T, Raison N, Haldar S, et al. Training tools for nontechnical skills for surgeons: a systematic review. J Surg Educ 2016;74(4):548–78.
76. Jamal M, Wong S, Whalen T. Effects of the reduction of surgical residents' work hours and implications for surgical residency programs: a narrative review. BMC Med Educ 2014;14:S14.
77. Mullen M, Salerno E, Michaels A, et al. Declining operative experience for junior-level residents: is this an unintended consequence of minimally invasive surgery? J Surg Educ 2016;73:609–15.
78. Willaert W, Aggarwal R, Van Herzeele I, et al. Recent advancements in medical simulation: patient-specific virtual reality simulation. World J Surg 2012;36:1703.
79. Cates C, Patel A, Nicholson W. Use of virtual reality simulation for mission rehearsal for carotid stenting. JAMA 2007;297:265–6.
80. Suzuki S, Eto K, Hattori A, et al. Surgery simulation using patient-specific models for laparoscopic colectomy. Stud Health Technol Inform 2007;125:464–6.
81. Weinstock P. Lifelike simulations that make real-life surgery safer. In: TEDxNatick. Available at: https://www.ted.com/talks/peter_weinstock_lifelike_simulations_that_make_real_life_surgery_safer. Accessed December 15, 2017.
82. Chalhoub E, Tanos V, Campo R. The role of video games in facilitating the psychomotor skills training in laparoscopic surgery. Gynecol Surg 2016;13:419–24.
83. Glassman D, Yiasemidou M, Ishii H, et al. Effect of playing video games on laparoscopic skills performance: a systematic review. J Endourol 2016;30(2):146–52.
84. El-Beheiry M, McCreey G, Schlachta C. A serious game skills competition increases voluntary usage and proficiency of a virtual reality laparoscopic simulator during first-year surgical residents' simulation curriculum. Surg Endosc 2017;31:1643–50.
85. Chang L, Petros J, Hess DT, et al. Integrating simulation into a surgical residency program: is voluntary participation effective? Surg Endosc 2007;21:418–21.
86. Ryan RM. The motivational pull of video games: a self-determination theory approach. Motiv Emot 2006;30:344–60.
87. Harbin A, Nadhan K, Mooney J. Prior video game utilization is associated with improved performance on a robotic skills simulator. J Robot Surg 2017;11:317–24.
88. Graafland M, Bemelman W, Schijven M. Game-based training improves the surgeon's situational awareness in the operation room: a randomized controlled trial. Surg Endosc 2017;31:4093–101.
89. Adams BJ, Margaron F, Kaplan BJ. Comparing video games and laparoscopic simulators in the development of laparoscopic skills in surgical residents. J Surg Educ 2012;69(6):714–7.
90. Hung A, Chen J, Shah A, et al. Telementoring and telesurgery for minimally invasive procedures. J Urol 2018;199:1–15.
91. Antoniou S, Antoniou G, Franzen J, et al. A comprehensive review of telementoring applications in laparoscopic general surgery. Surg Endosc 2012;26:2111–6.

Virtual and Augmented Reality in Oncologic Liver Surgery

Giuseppe Quero, MD[a], Alfonso Lapergola, MD[b], Luc Soler, PhD[b],
Jacques Marescaux, MD[a,b], Didier Mutter, MD, PhD[c],
Patrick Pessaux, MD, PhD[a,b,c],*

KEYWORDS

- Virtual reality • Augmented reality • Computer-assisted surgery
- Image-guided surgery • Precision surgery • Liver surgery
- 3-dimensional patient-specific modeling

KEY POINTS

- Imaging is a key factor in the evolution of precision surgery.
- Virtual reality software in surgery is the generation of 3-dimensional models of the patient's anatomy based on Digital Imaging and Communications in Medicine (DICOM) data of computed tomography or MRI scans.
- VR results in an interactive 3-dimensional environment, resulting in a realistic and immersive representation of a true-life experience.
- Augmented reality provides an enhanced rendering of VR to provide the surgeon with essential information to optimize navigation during complex surgery and to reduce intra- and postoperative complications.

INTRODUCTION

Imaging in general is a key component of the ongoing evolution of precision medicine, which is predicted to evolve tremendously through the use of big data and computer science. This evolution will provide automated and enhanced diagnostic and therapeutic algorithms.[1]

Disclosure: The institute IHU and IRCAD have funding by Storz, Siemens and Medtronic but not J Marescaux personally. Part of this research was financed by IRCAD and IHU, so indirectly by Storz, Siemens and Medtronic.

[a] IHU-Strasbourg, Institute of Image-Guided Surgery, 1 Place de l'Hôpital, Strasbourg 67091, France; [b] IRCAD, Research Institute Against Cancer of the Digestive System, 1 Place de l'Hôpital, Strasbourg 67091, France; [c] Department of General, Digestive and Endocrine Surgery, University Hospital of Strasbourg, 1 Place de l'Hôpital, Strasbourg 67091, France
* Corresponding author. 1, Place de l'Hôpital, Strasbourg 67091, France.
E-mail address: patrick.pessaux@ihu-strasbourg.eu

Surg Oncol Clin N Am 28 (2019) 31–44
https://doi.org/10.1016/j.soc.2018.08.002
1055-3207/19/© 2018 Elsevier Inc. All rights reserved.

surgonc.theclinics.com

This evolution is finding its way into surgery, especially complex interventions. In this context, hepatic surgery (HS) is particularly challenging due to its complex anatomy and intricate requirements for clinical decision making. Advanced imaging, such as virtual and augmented reality (AR), may help to overcome some of these challenges and optimize diagnosis and strategic therapeutic planning.[2]

Virtual reality (VR) is an interactive computer-generated 3-dimensional environment, allowing for a realistic and immersive experience. Applied to medicine, VR software generates 3-dimensional models of patients that are based on Digital Imaging and Communications in Medicine (DICOM) data of computed tomography (CT) or MRI scans. Most radiologic workstations can provide the patient-specific anatomy in a 3-dimensional format using direct volume rendering (DVR). Volumetric medical image rendering is a method of extracting important information from a 3-dimensional dataset, allowing a better understanding of disease processes and anatomy. However, it does not enable interactive modeling of individual organs[3] and is therefore not suitable for computer-assisted surgery. More specifically, organs can neither be manipulated individually within the virtual environment to facilitate a surgical approach nor modeled to augment the 3-dimensional environment. Although DVR has challenges regarding its use in computer-assisted surgery. its advantage is easy usability. In this context, DVR is available on personal computers thanks to open-source software such as Slicer,[4] Osirix on MacOS,[5] VR RENDER and VR-Planning[6] on Windows, MacOS, and Linux.

In contrast to DVR, surface rendering (SR) is a process requiring 3-dimensional virtual modeling of the patients' organs (also known as organ delineation or segmentation). SR involves reconstructing 3-dimensional geometric meshes of the organ surfaces through manual, semiautomatic, or fully automatic software processes. Thereby, SR enables the manipulation of a virtual representation of the patient. Zooming, rotating with all degrees of freedom, and application of modular virtual transparency of different organs are possible. The difference in rendering between DVR and SR is depicted in **Fig. 1**.

The next step in the development of AR is the combination of VR and SR. Combining VR with SR enables a deep understanding of the anatomy and can

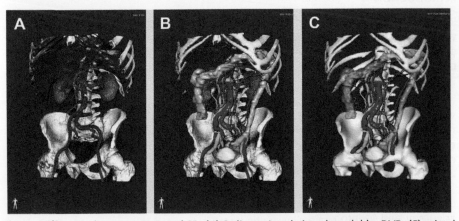

Fig. 1. Difference between DVR and SR. (*A*) 3-dimensional virtual model by DVR, (*B*) mixed view by DVR with SR segmented structures (vessels, urinary bladder, ureters, and colon), and (*C*) SR view (the segmented organs can be individually manipulated and selectively removed to improve the navigation).

show anatomic variants and complex anatomic relationships that may be missed on conventional DICOM imaging.[7,8] The resulting patient model enables a virtual surgical exploration, development of a detailed patient-specific preoperative surgical plan, and simulation of both surgery or ablation approaches.[9] For HS specifically, AR provides an accurate computation of liver volume, preoperative planning of resection planes along liver segments, optimal targeting of portal pedicles, and analysis of tumor margins.

The authors have developed software solutions for creating patient-specific models and SR visualizations that have been applied to various clinical scenarios, including endocrine surgery,[10] transanal total mesorectal excision,[11] and hepatobiliary surgery.[12–15] As mentioned earlier, VR cannot only be used for preoperative planning but also during the surgical procedure to provide surgical navigation. In this context, the authors have combined SR and VR to perform AR navigation. AR is defined as the superimposition of virtual images of organs (generated by SR) on actual intraoperative images. An important feature of advanced AR is the possibility to hide or accentuate organs using a specific modular transparency function.[2,16]

How is AR projected onto the patient's anatomy so that if the view of the surgeon changes or organs are moved, the AR is still superimposed accurately? Registration is the process of overlying the 3-dimensional virtual images to the real-time operative images of the patient. This process can be manual, semiautomated, or fully automated. In the first case, the preoperative 3-dimensional model is displayed on the operative monitor and manually oriented and/or resized to fit the real images. The semiautomatic method requires landmark structures to be identified on the 3-dimensional model and on the operative image. Then the AR is manually overlaid onto the real-life images using these landmarks known as registration. Following registration, various methods of automated tracking of these landmarks are used to reposition the 3-dimensional virtual model as the real-life images move.[17] The process is semiautomated, because registration is manual, while the tracking is automated. The precision of the 3-dimensional virtual tracking technique (manual vs semiautomatic) is a critical factor of the resected volume and can be measured. The semiautomatic method using the actual resected specimen for confirmation has been shown to be more precise than a manual method.[18]

Fully automatic registration remains a major challenge today and is subject to ongoing research.[19–21] These challenges are due to the difficulty of obtaining an accurate and real-time automatic registration in soft tissue surgery. Soft tissues such as the liver are subject to organ motion and deformation because of respiration, pneumoperitoneum, and/or surgical manipulation. This leads to inaccuracies of registration and subsequent imprecise overlap of 3-dimensional virtual images and real-life images.

The augmented information is displayed to the surgical team in various formats for various surgical approaches (Fig. 2). In this context, it has been successfully applied to not only open surgery but also minimally invasive laparoscopic and robotic liver resections. These seem to benefit particularly from AR applications due to the innate technical challenges of minimally invasive surgery such as reduced haptic feedback and limits of the visual field.[19–21]

Here is provided an overview of state-of-the-art VR- and AR-guided hepatobiliary oncologic surgery. The focus lies on the ability of these technologies to increase accuracy and to inform the surgeon during preoperative and intraoperative decision making. Reports included in this article include the number of patients and the clinical diagnosis for which AR or VR was applied; these are summarized in **Table 1**.

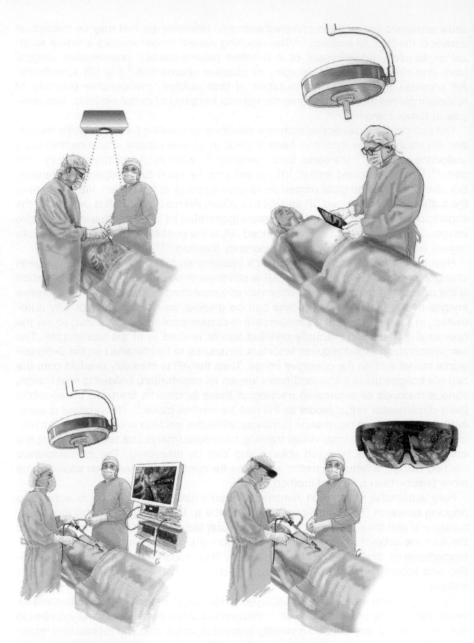

Fig. 2. AR display methods. (*Upper row*) The virtual model can be directly projected on the patient anatomy using a projector beam, or it can be visualized using calibrated see-through devices. (*Lower row*) The VR model can also be visualized on the screen in camera-based AR, during minimally invasive procedures, or using goggle head-mounted devices.

Virtual Reality

Today, virtual reality for the application in surgery and in particular HS is an area of active research. Seventeen studies on the use of VR in liver surgery (total of 740 patients) have been published. The application of 3-dimensional virtual reality in these articles is predominantly to plan and preoperatively simulate a liver interventions. Malignancy was the indication for VR reconstruction in 546 cases (73.7%), mainly for hepatocellular carcinoma (HCC, 303 cases), followed by colorectal cancer liver metastasis (CRLM;,198 cases). Surgical resection was successfully performed in 622 patients through open access and in 36 cases via a laparoscopic approach. In 1 case series that included 20 patients,[30] VR was used to plan and perform transarterial chemoembolization. The software used in these studies significantly varied among the studies.

A key factor in making 3-dimensional VR clinically applicable is cutting down on time and effort required to create a patient-specific VR. The 3-dimensional virtual modeling time has been reported in 4 studies only[23,29,30,34] and significantly varied according to the software characteristics. The mean value of VR creation time has become significantly faster over time and has been reported as a mean of 32.1 minutes (range 5.1–75 minutes).

Accuracy for 3-dimensional VR is defined as the relative difference between calculated liver volume and volume of the actual liver resection.[18,22,26,27,29,34,36] Yamanaka and colleagues[34] compared the predicted resection volumes with the weight of the specimen obtained. Additionally, a comparison between liver resection volume in the 3-dimensional simulation and the preoperative planimetry was carried out. Moreover, the investigators compared the resection margins in cancer cases at risk for a positive margin as predicted at time of VR simulation with the actual histopathologic margin status. In major and minor hepatectomies, a high correlation was reported between the simulated resection weight and actual weight (r: 0.96). The same group[27] had recently reported similar results in laparoscopic hepatectomies in a cohort of 35 patients. The differences between VR and specimen were a low liver volume difference of 21 plus or minus 44.6 mL (r: 0.995) and a margin difference of 1.3 plus or minus 4.8 mm (r: 0.702). The authors and colleagues reported not only on cancer resection. A cohort of 106 patients affected by hepatic alveolar echinococcosis underwent preoperative virtual 3-dimensional liver resection (59 patients) or conventional imaging methods (47 patients).[22] The estimated resection of liver volumes in both groups had good correlation with the specimen weight obtained, with an r value of 0.98 for the 3-dimensional reconstruction group and r: 0.96 in the conventional imaging group. Similar comparisons with high correlations in terms of calculated liver and tumor volume and the actual ones have been reported.[26,29,36]

VR has not only been evaluated regarding its accuracy in registration or liver volume prediction, but also its ability to provide critical information that may change the surgical strategy. Tian and colleagues[26] reported changes in the surgical management in 2 cases following the application of 3-dimensional VR. In a patient with a large HCC at the drainage of the right and middle hepatic vein into the IVC, standard imaging was deemed insufficient to judge operability. However, 3-dimensional VR planning favored surgical resection, which was successfully performed. In a second case of HCC of the left lobe, a left hepatectomy was considered feasible on conventional CT scan and ultrasound, but the 3-dimensinal VR planning revealed tumor infiltration into the middle hepatic vein, leading the surgeons to perform a mesohepatectomy including the middle hepatic vein.

Similarly, VR demonstrated its value in the series[34] of HCC cases in patients with impaired liver function. An example of the value of VR to prevent postoperative liver failure is 3-dimensional virtual modeling leading to the recognition of a right and middle aberrant hepatic vein subsequently avoiding improper outflow resection and risk for postoperative liver failure.[35] Change in surgical evaluation from unresectable to

Table 1
Study characteristics

Author, Year	Number of Patients	Hepatic Disease		Software	3-Dimensional VR Reconstruction Time (min)	Accuracy	
		Malignant	Others			Volume	Margins
Virtual reality							
He et al,[22] 2015	106	—	106	IQQA-Liver	—	0.98	—
Su et al,[23] 2016	26	—	26	Hisense CAS	30	—	—
Xiang et al,[24] 2015	1	1	—	MI-3DVS	—	—	—
Su et al,[25] 2015	21	13	8	Higemi	—	—	—
Tian et al,[26] 2015	39	39	—	Yorktal DMIT	—	—	—
Bégin et al,[18] 2014	43	34	9	VR-RENDER	—	0.758	—
Yamanaka et al,[27] 2009	113	113	—	Hitachi Image Processing System	75	0.96a	0.84
Mutter et al,[13] 2009	1	1	—	VD-RENDER	—	—	—
Xie et al,[28] 2013	20	—	20	FreeForm Modeling System	—	—	—
Takamoto et al,[29] 2013	83	83	—	Synapse VINCENT	18.3	0.99	—
Bargellini et al,[30] 2013	20	20	—	Innova Vision	5.1	—	—
Radtke et al,[31] 2010	202	183	19	HepaVision 3D-CASP	—	—	—
Oldhafer et al,[32] 2009	1	1	—	MeVis	—	—	—

					Registration		
					Mode	Time (min)	Accuracy (mm)
Endo et al,[33] 2007	1	1	—	HepaVision	—	—	—
Yamanaka et al,[34] 2007	35	32	3	Organs Volume Analysis		0.995	0.702
Lang et al,[35] 2004	1	1	—	MeVis		—	—
Wigmore et al,[36] 2001	27	26	1	GE Advantage Windows		0.97	—
Augmented Reality							
Ntourakis et al,[37] 2016	3	3	—	VR-RENDER	Manual	5	5
Hallet et al,[21] 2015	1	1	—	VR-RENDER	Manual	—	—
Pessaux et al,[20] 2015	3	2	1	VR-RENDER	Manual	8	—
Kenngott et al,[38] 2014	1	1	—	Syngo iPilot	Semiautomatic	—	0.93
Onda et al,[39] 2013	2	2	—	Analyze	Manual and semiautomatic	1.5	10.59
Buchs et al,[40] 2013	2	2	—	MeVis	Automatic	2	—
Okamoto et al,[41] 2013	3	2	1	Analyze	Semiautomatic	—	5
Souzaki et al,[42] 2013	1	—	1	Virtual Place 300	Semiautomatic	—	—

Only patients with liver and biliary diseases were included; volumes and margin evaluated in terms of r value. Only studies with r value are reported.
[a] Only major hepatectomies were evaluated.

resectable has also been shown in pediatric surgery applications of VR.[23] An extreme demonstration on change of surgical strategy[31] has been reported when 67% of cases changed from resectable to unresectable by preoperative 3-dimensional virtual modeling and VR compared with classical 2-dimensional scan analysis. Further, in the cases where actual surgical resection was possible, 3-dimensional VR influenced the surgical strategy in one-third of the cases, extending resection and adding intra-hepatic vascular reconstruction in 53 cases. In 3 cases, the 3-dimensional simulation led to a radically different surgical strategy compared with the proposed 2-dimensioal strategy.

Despite the overall low level of evidence of the published literature regarding the contribution of 3-dimensional VR to surgery today, VR planning has been reported as an important method in predicting resected liver volume compared with standard imaging. In addition, authors agree on the utility of VR reconstruction in performing highly complex surgical procedures with important implications on decision making regarding resectability and choice of operative strategy.

Augmented Reality

AR-assisted surgery is a surgical tool utilizing technology that superimposes a computer-generated enhanced image on a surgeon's view of the operative field, thus providing a composite view. This composite view for the surgeon is provided by a computer-generated overlay with the goal of improving the operative experi-ence. All investigators who have used AR report an increased accuracy in tumor localization and resection as well as a significantly more precise understanding of vascular anatomy. In HS application, various tumor types have been resected under AR guidance including HCC, CRLM, cholangiocarcinoma, gallbladder cancer, and hepatoblastoma.

A particular application of AR guidance has been reported by Ntourakis and colleagues[37] in the treatment of disappearing CRLM after chemotherapy. A 3-dimen-sional virtual model of the patient's liver was created before and after chemotherapy. In the case of disappearing metastases, the prechemotherapy patient model was pro-jected onto the postchemotherapy model. Consequently, all the metastases evident on the preoperative images were superimposed to the intraoperative real-time im-ages. Thereby, all sites of missing metastases were identified through AR guidance and successfully resected. The clinical importance of resecting disappearing CRLM was confirmed by the presence of residual cancer tissue at the site of some lesions.

The accuracy of registration of AR to the patient-specific anatomy remains a chal-lenge. Today, intraoperative ultrasound (IOUS) is being used to confirm the accuracy of registration of the AR.[20,21,41] The 3-dimensional virtual models were obtained us-ing different software with the goal of reducing discrepancy between true patient anatomy and the AR.[20,21,37] This is a particular challenge in minimally invasive sur-gery, where pneumoperitoneum at time of surgery leads to inaccurate registration. However, modelling has been developed to overcome this challenge as demon-strated in 3 robotic hepatic segmentectomies, allowing the prediction of the final po-sition of organs and abdominal wall after peritoneal insufflation at a constant pneumoperitoneal pressure of 12 mm Hg. In all reported series,[20,21,37] the registra-tion was performed manually. However, semiautomatic AR registration approaches are developing. For example, semiautomatic registration has been used[38] using intraoperative C-arm cone-beam CT images which were correlated to preoperative MRI images for the detection of difficult to visualize tumors. Onda and colleagues[39] performed registration semiautomatically by measuring the position of anatomic landmarks through tracking 24 infrared-omitting diode markers (Optotrack pen probe). The achieved AR navigation accuracy has been reported to lie within a mean error of 5.38 mm (0.93–10.59 mm).[37–39,41,42] To improve the accuracy of AR registration in open surgery, respiratory gaiting has been used. For example, to minimize the registration error, AR guidance was performed only in the expiratory phase, with an accuracy of 5 mm.[37] Another approach to improve accuracy in robotic surgery is to measure the precision of image superimposition, using surface (lower costal edge, iliac crest, and umbilicus) and intraabdominal landmarks (inferior vena cava and robotic tools).[20] Another technique is using the tumor and a gating clip as registration landmarks during the superimposition phase.[38] This can result in an accuracy estimated preoperatively on a phantom model of 0.93 mm. Despite registration errors in all included studies, the resection margin proved to be negative in all reported cases. The total time required to obtain AR guidance (registration time) ranged between 1 and 8 minutes (mean value 4.1 minutes) without an impact on total operation time.[20,37,39,40] Although the results of the reported studies are promising, intraoperative deformation from manipulation of the operative field by the surgeon has not modeled and remains a significant challenge limiting clinical applicability. (**Fig. 3**)

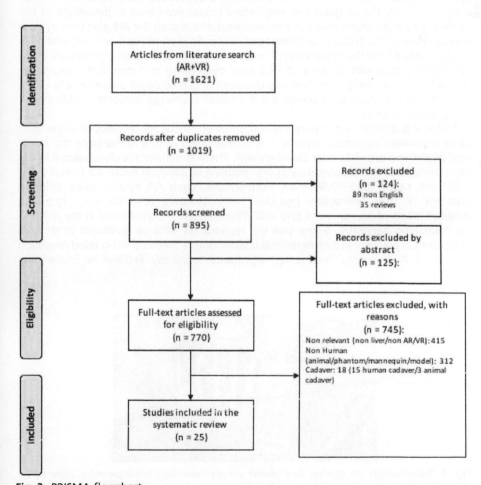

Fig. 3. PRISMA flowchart.

DISCUSSION

The creation of 3-dimensional virtual models of patient anatomy from preoperative images (VR-based strategy) may help surgeons with preoperative planning[32,43] and to reduce procedure-related complications.[44] The need for precise modeling when assessing the size of the functional liver remnant is particularly important when performing major liver resection. In this context, the use of VR modeling has been demonstrated to be accurate, reliable, and efficient.[13,20,45,46] A particular important application may be the use of AR navigation to identify disappearing colorectal metastasis following neoadjuvant chemotherapy.[32,37] Further, although not discussed here, AR may become an important component of surgical training, procedure standardization, and surgical access planning.[47] In this context, AR has been shown to be helpful in surgical access planning for challenging MIS HS. In a difficult case of a patient with a tumor at the liver dome, AR guidance was successfully used to guide a transthoracic minimally invasive resection[21] (**Fig. 4**).

The key aspect governing the efficacy of an AR system is accuracy, reliability, and repeatability of its registration process. Because the 3-dimensional virtual model is a only preoperative static snapshot of a specific preoperative body position,[15,48] liver manipulation by the surgeon and respiratory movements lead to deviations of the modeling from the static preoperative snapshot and impact the AR guidance system performance. In the authors' experience of AR application where liver manipulation is not accounted for in the registration process, maximum registration error occurs in the inspiratory phase with an error of 13.3 mm, decreasing to 5 mm in the expiratory phase.[37,49,50] Accounting for liver manipulation and predicable displacement of organs during the respiratory phase are the major challenge preventing widespread AR application today.

Today, it is difficult to compare the outcomes of various AR techniques in the literature for several important reasons. It is a developing field, and therefore standardized algorithms are still under development. There is substantial discrepancy in the algorithms used and discrepancy in the reported registration accuracy (mean value 5.38 mm, range 0.93–10.59 mm). Furthermore, each AR system uses different amounts of user interaction (manual, semiautomatic, or automatic), requiring different levels of human input and skill. There is also inconsistency in the method for measuring accuracy. Some use the registration error at anatomic landmarks (measured in pixels or in 3-dimensional space); others measure AR-guided resection margins.[40] Furthermore, measuring registration accuracy in itself is challenging (**Fig. 5**).

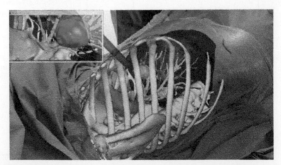

Fig. 4. Transthoracic AR-guided liver dome cancer resection. Intraoperative view of an AR-guided liver dome cancer resection by transthoracic approach.

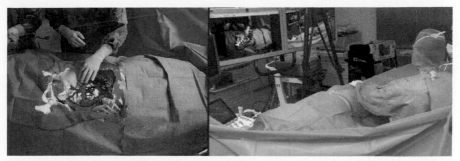

Fig. 5. AR-guided visualization dedicated to liver radiofrequency ablation. The 3-dimensional virtual modeling is registered via a nonrigid approach taking change in patient position accurately into account.

Few patients have been operated using AR technologies to date. The main reasons are that AR with soft tissue surgery is highly challenging and has limits regarding the accuracy of virtual model registration. Nevertheless, many surgical laboratories dedicated to computer-assisted surgery are actively working on improving the AR reliability. Promising approaches to overcome registration errors are predictive real-time simulation of organ deformation during breathing.[51,52] Among other solutions towards improving registration accuracy, the authors are working on the use of near-infrared fluorescence technologies. The intensity of the fluorescent signal emitted from fluorescent markers placed on the surface of organs may allow a robust registration of the VR model on real-time camera images.[53]

Another future trend is the incorporation of complementary intraoperative imaging modalities. Shekhar and colleagues[54] have proposed using a low-dose intraoperative CT scan together with an optical tracking system that trails the endoscopic camera to update the 3-dimensional reconstruction. This approach, however, provides less detailed AR images than can be achieved with standard preoperative CT images. Further, others have proposed a 3-dimensional image acquisition method using 3-dimensional ultrasound.[55] In this context, the authors are working on a 4-dimensional ultrasound probe, enabling image fusion of CT and MRI with real-time ultrasonography.

In conclusion, despite the current limitations, the use of VR and AR navigation systems has shown a potential clinical utility, especially in cases of complex liver surgery. Preoperative simulation of the surgical procedure and accurate user-friendly calculation of the future liver remnant can significantly decrease improper surgical procedures and postoperative complications. Moreover, AR navigation facilitates recognition and localization of anatomic structures. The goal of achieving fully automated, robust, reproducible, and rapidly updated soft tissue AR registration is the next step towards the more widespread clinical application for a safer and more precise surgery.

REFERENCES

1. Collins FS, Varmus H. A new initiative on precision medicine. N Engl J Med 2015; 372:793–5.
2. Marescaux J, Diana M. Inventing the future of surgery. World J Surg 2015;39: 615–22.
3. Calhoun PS, Kuszyk BS, Heath DG, et al. Three-dimensional volume rendering of spiral CT data: theory and method. Radiographics 1999;19:745–04.

4. Fedorov A, Beichel R, Kalpathy-Cramer J, et al. 3D Slicer as an Image Computing Platform for the Quantitative Imaging Network. Magn Reson Imaging 2012;30(9): 1323–41.

5. Volonte F, Pugin F, Bucher P, et al. Augmented reality and image overlay navigation with OsiriX in laparoscopic and robotic surgery: not only a matter of fashion. J Hepatobiliary Pancreat Sci 2011;18:506–9.

6. Nicolau S, Soler L, Mutter D, et al. Augmented reality in laparoscopic surgical oncology. Surg Oncol 2011;20:189–201.

7. D'Agostino J, Diana M, Vix M, et al. Three-dimensional virtual neck exploration before parathyroidectomy. N Engl J Med 2012;367:1072–3.

8. Diana M, Soler L, Agnus V, et al. Prospective evaluation of precision multimodal gallbladder surgery navigation: virtual reality, near-infrared fluorescence, and X-ray-based intraoperative cholangiography. Ann Surg 2017;266(5):890–7.

9. Soler L, Delingette H, Malandain G, et al. An automatic virtual patient reconstruction from CT-scans for hepatic surgical planning. Stud Health Technol Inform 2000;70:316–22.

10. D'Agostino J, Diana M, Vix M, et al. Three-dimensional metabolic and radiologic gathered evaluation using VR-RENDER fusion: a novel tool to enhance accuracy in the localization of parathyroid adenomas. World J Surg 2013;37:1618–25.

11. Franchini Melani AG, Diana M, Marescaux J. The quest for precision in transanal total mesorectal excision. Tech Coloproctol 2016;20:11–8.

12. Marescaux J, Clement JM, Tassetti V, et al. Virtual reality applied to hepatic surgery simulation: the next revolution. Ann Surg 1998;228:627–34.

13. Mutter D, Dallemagne B, Bailey C, et al. 3D virtual reality and selective vascular control for laparoscopic left hepatic lobectomy. Surg Endosc 2009;23:432–5.

14. Simone M, Mutter D, Rubino F, et al. Three-dimensional virtual cholangioscopy: a reliable tool for the diagnosis of common bile duct stones. Ann Surg 2004;240: 82–8.

15. Soler L, Nicolau S, Pessaux P, et al. Real-time 3D image reconstruction guidance in liver resection surgery. Hepatobiliary Surg Nutr 2014;3:73–81.

16. Marescaux J, Rubino F, Arenas M, et al. Augmented-reality-assisted laparoscopic adrenalectomy. JAMA 2004;292:2214–5.

17. Marvik R, Lango T, Tangen GA, et al. Laparoscopic navigation pointer for three-dimensional image-guided surgery. Surg Endosc 2004;18:1242–8.

18. Bégin A, Martel G, Lapointe R, et al. Accuracy of preoperative automatic measurement of the liver volume by CT-scan combined to a 3D virtual surgical planning software (3DVSP). Surg Endosc 2014;28:3408–12.

19. Mutter D, Soler L, Marescaux J. Recent advances in liver imaging. Expert Rev Gastroenterol Hepatol 2010;4:613–21.

20. Pessaux P, Diana M, Soler L, et al. Towards cybernetic surgery: robotic and augmented reality-assisted liver segmentectomy. Langenbecks Arch Surg 2015;400:381–5.

21. Hallet J, Soler L, Diana M, et al. Trans-thoracic minimally invasive liver resection guided by augmented reality. J Am Coll Surg 2015;220:e55–60.

22. He YB, Bai L, Aji T, et al. Application of 3D reconstruction for surgical treatment of hepatic alveolar echinococcosis. World J Gastroenterol 2015;21:10200–7.

23. Su L, Dong Q, Zhang H, et al. Clinical application of a three-dimensional imaging technique in infants and young children with complex liver tumors. Pediatr Surg Int 2016;32:387–95.

24. Xiang N, Fang C, Fan Y, et al. Application of liver three-dimensional printing in hepatectomy for complex massive hepatocarcinoma with rare variations of portal vein: preliminary experience. Int J Clin Exp Med 2015;8:18873–8.

25. Su L, Zhou XJ, Dong Q, et al. Application value of computer assisted surgery system in precision surgeries for pediatric complex liver tumors. Int J Clin Exp Med 2015;8:18406–12.

26. Tian F, Wu JX, Rong WQ, et al. Three-dimensional morphometric analysis for hepatectomy of centrally located hepatocellular carcinoma: a pilot study. World J Gastroenterol 2015;21:4607–19.

27. Yamanaka J, Okada T, Saito S, et al. Minimally invasive laparoscopic liver resection: 3D MDCT simulation for preoperative planning. J Hepatobiliary Pancreat Sci 2009;16:808–15.

28. Xie A, Fang C, Huang Y, et al. Application of three-dimensional reconstruction and visible simulation technique in reoperation of hepatolithiasis. J Gastroenterol Hepatol 2013;28:248–54.

29. Takamoto T, Hashimoto T, Ogata S, et al. Planning of anatomical liver segmentectomy and subsegmentectomy with 3-dimensional simulation software. Am J Surg 2013;206:530–8.

30. Bargellini I, Turini F, Bozzi E, et al. Image fusion of preprocedural CTA with real-time fluoroscopy to guide proper hepatic artery catheterization during transarterial chemoembolization of hepatocellular carcinoma: a feasibility study. Cardiovasc Intervent Radiol 2013;36:526–30.

31. Radtke A, Sotiropoulos GC, Molmenti EP, et al. Computer-assisted surgery planning for complex liver resections: when is it helpful? A single-center experience over an 8-year period. Ann Surg 2010;252:876–83.

32. Oldhafer KJ, Stavrou GA, Prause G, et al. How to operate a liver tumor you cannot see. Langenbecks Arch Surg 2009;394:489–94.

33. Endo I, Shimada H, Takeda K, et al. Successful duct-to-duct biliary reconstruction after right hemihepatectomy. Operative planning using virtual 3D reconstructed images. J Gastrointest Surg 2007;11:666–70.

34. Yamanaka J, Saito S, Fujimoto J. Impact of preoperative planning using virtual segmental volumetry on liver resection for hepatocellular carcinoma. World J Surg 2007;31:1249–55.

35. Lang H, Radtke A, Liu C, et al. Extended left hepatectomy–modified operation planning based on three-dimensional visualization of liver anatomy. Langenbeck's Arch Surg 2004;389:306–10.

36. Wigmore SJ, Redhead DN, Yan XJ, et al. Virtual hepatic resection using three-dimensional reconstruction of helical computed tomography angioportograms. Ann Surg 2001;233:221–6.

37. Ntourakis D, Memeo R, Soler L, et al. Augmented reality guidance for the resection of missing colorectal liver metastases: an initial experience. World J Surg 2016;40:419–26.

38. Kenngott HG, Wagner M, Gondan M, et al. Real-time image guidance in laparoscopic liver surgery: first clinical experience with a guidance system based on intraoperative CT imaging. Surg Endosc 2014;28:933–40.

39. Onda S, Okamoto T, Kanehira M, et al. Short rigid scope and stereo-scope designed specifically for open abdominal navigation surgery: clinical application for hepatobiliary and pancreatic surgery. J Hepatobiliary Pancreat Sci 2013;20:448–53.

40. Buchs NC, Volonte F, Pugin F, et al. Augmented environments for the targeting of hepatic lesions during image-guided robotic liver surgery. J Surg Res 2013;184: 825–31.
41. Okamoto T, Onda S, Matsumoto M, et al. Utility of augmented reality system in hepatobiliary surgery. J Hepatobiliary Pancreat Sci 2013;20:249–53.
42. Souzaki R, Ieiri S, Uemura M, et al. An augmented reality navigation system for pediatric oncologic surgery based on preoperative CT and MRI images. J Pediatr Surg 2013;48:2479–83.
43. Herfarth C, Lamade W, Fischer L, et al. The effect of virtual reality and training on liver operation planning. Swiss Surg 2002;8:67–73.
44. Chen G, Li XC, Wu GQ, et al. The use of virtual reality for the functional simulation of hepatic tumors (case control study). Int J Surg 2010;8:72–8.
45. Marzano E, Piardi T, Soler L, et al. Augmented reality-guided artery-first pancreatico-duodenectomy. J Gastrointest Surg 2013;17:1980–3.
46. Pessaux P, Diana M, Soler L, et al. Robotic duodenopancreatectomy assisted with augmented reality and real-time fluorescence guidance. Surg Endosc 2014;28:2493–8.
47. Vera AM, Russo M, Mohsin A, et al. Augmented reality telementoring (ART) platform: a randomized controlled trial to assess the efficacy of a new surgical education technology. Surg Endosc 2014;28:3467–72.
48. Bernhardt S, Nicolau SA, Soler L, et al. The status of augmented reality in laparoscopic surgery as of 2016. Med Image Anal 2017;37:66–90.
49. Nicolau SA, Pennec X, Soler L, et al. Clinical evaluation of a respiratory gated guidance system for liver punctures. Med Image Comput Comput Assist Interv 2007;10:77–85.
50. Hostettler A, Nicolau SA, Remond Y, et al. A real-time predictive simulation of abdominal viscera positions during quiet free breathing. Prog Biophys Mol Biol 2010;103:169–84.
51. Haouchine N, Dequidt J, Berger MO, et al. Deformation-based augmented reality for hepatic surgery. Stud Health Technol Inform 2013;184:182–8.
52. Umale S, Chatelin S, Bourdet N, et al. Experimental in vitro mechanical characterization of porcine Glisson's capsule and hepatic veins. J Biomech 2011;44: 1678–83.
53. Kong SH, Haouchine N, Soares R, et al. Robust augmented reality registration method for localization of solid organs' tumors using CT-derived virtual biomechanical model and fluorescent fiducials. Surg Endosc 2016;31(7):2863–71.
54. Shekhar R, Dandekar O, Bhat V, et al. Live augmented reality: a new visualization method for laparoscopic surgery using continuous volumetric computed tomography. Surg Endosc 2010;24:1976–85.
55. Nam WH, Kang DG, Lee D, et al. Automatic registration between 3D intraoperative ultrasound and pre-operative CT images of the liver based on robust edge matching. Phys Med Biol 2012;57:69–91.

Fluorescence Imaging for Minimally Invasive Cancer Surgery

Takeaki Ishizawa, MD, PhD*, Akio Saiura, MD, PhD

KEYWORDS

- Fluorescence imaging • Intraoperative cholangiography • Liver cancer
- Pancreatic cancer • Indocyanine green

KEY POINTS

- The basis of indocyanine green fluorescence imaging is that protein-bound indocyanine green emits fluorescence signals when illuminated with near-infrared light.
- To identify liver cancer, indocyanine green is injected intravenously approximately 2 weeks before surgery. Administration of indocyanine green the day before surgery should be avoided to decrease the incidence of false-positive nodules.
- In fluorescence cholangiography, indocyanine green is injected intravenously at least 15 minutes before detection; the optimal time of injection is approximately 90 minutes before observation.
- Five to 10 mL of indocyanine green solution diluted to a concentration of 0.05 to 0.25 mg/mL is injected into the segmental portal branch under ultrasound guidance for the delineation of hepatic segments. Alternatively, indocyanine green can be injected intravenously after closure of the corresponding portal pedicle.
- Real-time fluorescence images of vascular structures are obtained after intravenous bolus injection of indocyanine green, preferably from a central venous catheter.

INTRODUCTION

One of the major difficulties of minimally invasive cancer surgery lies in understanding the extent of cancerous tissues and its surrounding anatomic structures. This is due to limitations in palpation and surgical view as compared with open surgery. Traditionally, intraoperative ultrasound imaging and radiographic angiography/cholangiography have been used for the identification of anatomic structures in digestive surgery. However, it can be challenging to understand the spatial relationship between

Disclosure: This work was supported by grants from the Foundation for Promotion of Cancer Research and the Japanese Foundation for Research and Promotion of Endoscopy, Japan.
Department of Gastroenterological Surgery, Cancer Institute Hospital, Japanese Foundation for Cancer Research, 3-8-31 Ariake, Koto-ku, Tokyo 135-8655, Japan
* Corresponding author.
E-mail address: tish-tky@umin.ac.jp

tumors and critical anatomic structures, especially during laparoscopic or robot-assisted surgery when only conventional imaging modalities are available.

The recent development of in vivo fluorescence imaging techniques using indocyanine green (ICG) as the main fluorogenic reagent, allows for the real-time visualization of cancerous tissues and anatomic structures.[1] After ICG was first approved by the US Food and Drug Administration in 1954, it was applied clinically first to estimate cardiac output and liver function. It was not until later that the fluorescence property of ICG was characterized in detail: protein-bound ICG emits fluorescence that peaks at around 840 nm when illuminated with near-infrared light (750–810 nm).[2] Because this wavelength is barely absorbed by hemoglobin or water, structures that contain ICG can be visualized by a near-infrared camera system through human tissue with a thicknesses of up to 5 to 10 mm. In hepatobiliary surgery, ICG fluorescence imaging can be used to delineate bile duct anatomy, hepatic tumors, and boundaries of hepatic segments. In this context, the differential ability between tumors and normal liver to excrete ICG via bile (tumor detection) and the fluorescence property of ICG when used for positive or negative staining (anatomy delineation) make it a powerful diagnostic modality. Herein, the authors provide a practical description of ICG fluorescence imaging techniques of minimally invasive surgery with a special focus on its applications in laparoscopic hepatobiliary and pancreatic surgery.

SURGICAL TECHNIQUE
Preoperative Planning

Applications of ICG fluorescence imaging in hepatobiliary and pancreatic surgery include (i) liver cancer identification, (ii) fluorescence cholangiography, (iii) delineation of hepatic segments, and (iv) fluorescence angiography and perfusion assessment. The timing of ICG injection is a critical factor for optimal usage. For example, fluorescence imaging of hepatic tumors requires preoperative intravenous administration of ICG. This procedure is also recommended to obtain clear fluorescence images of the bile ducts with a high signal-to-background contrast. Conversely, intraoperative administration of ICG shortly before bile duct visualization is used for fluorescence cholangiography.

As mentioned, the identification of hepatic tumors by intraoperative fluorescence imaging, requires intravenous injection of ICG before surgery.[3] Although the optimal dose and timing of ICG injection for primary liver cancer imaging have not been clearly determined yet,[4] the authors usually administer ICG at a dose of 0.5 mg/kg of the patient's body weight within 2 weeks before surgery. In this context of preoperative ICG administration, the primary use is for the preoperative evaluation of liver function. After ICG administration, ICG accumulates in cancerous tissues of well-differentiated hepatocellular carcinoma, noncancerous hepatic parenchyma surrounding poorly differentiated hepatocellular carcinoma, adenocarcinomas such as colorectal liver metastasis, and intrahepatic cholangiocarcinoma (**Fig. 1**). This preoperative administration enables intraoperative visualization of subcapsular hepatic tumors by fluorescence imaging.[3,5,6] Administration of ICG on the day before surgery should be avoided to decrease the incidence of false-positive lesions, especially in patients with decreased liver function owing to hepatitis/cirrhosis or preoperative chemotherapy.

Regarding intraoperative fluorescence cholangiography, the authors have found that a time interval of 90 minutes or greater between preoperative ICG administration (2.5 mg) and subsequent fluorescence imaging to visualized the bile duct is optimal.[7] In patients undergoing hepatectomy after a preoperative ICG retention test, fluorescence imaging often enables visualization of the extrahepatic bile duct anatomy

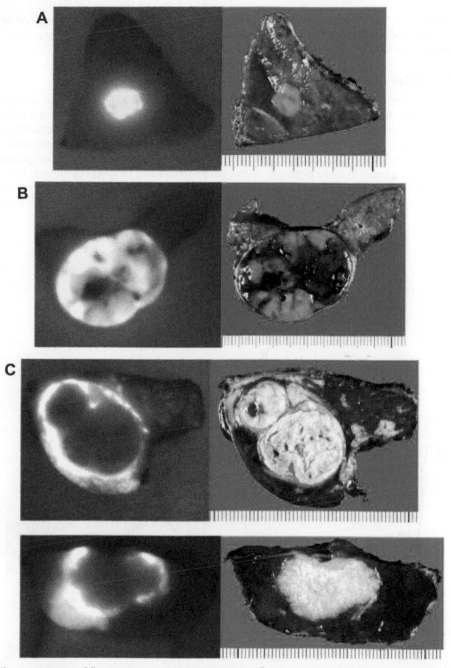

Fig. 1. Patterns of fluorescence signals in liver cancer. On the cut surfaces of liver cancers, patterns of fluorescence signals following preoperative intravenous injection of indocyanine green can be classified into a total fluorescence type (*A*, well-differentiated hepatocellular carcinoma [HCC]), a partial fluorescence type (*B*, moderately differentiated HCC), and a rim fluorescence type (*C*, poorly differentiated HCC [*upper*] and colorectal liver metastasis [*lower*]). (*From* Ishizawa T, Harada N, Muraoka A, et al. Scientific basis and clinical application of ICG fluorescence imaging: hepatobiliary cancer. Open Surg Oncol J 2010;2:34; with permission.)

without additional injection of ICG for cholangiography. The reason is that excretion of ICG into the bile can last for several days after the intravenous injection for preoperative liver function testing (of the conventional dose of 0.5 mg/kg).[8]

Preparation and Patient Positioning

Patients are placed in the French position (lithotomy with the legs spread and bent at the knees). For a standard laparoscopic hepatectomy, 5 trocars are placed in the right upper quadrant of the abdomen (**Fig. 2A**).[9] In patients with hepatic tumors located in segments 7 and/or 8, 1 or 2 balloon-tipped trocars are deployed through the intercostal space and the diaphragm (intercostal trocars). This access enables surgeons to identify tumors in close proximity to the laparoscope and to keep the hepatic transection planes vertical to the hepatic surface. Additionally, minimal mobilization of the right liver is required (**Fig. 2B**).[9,10] For identification of subphrenic hepatic tumors by

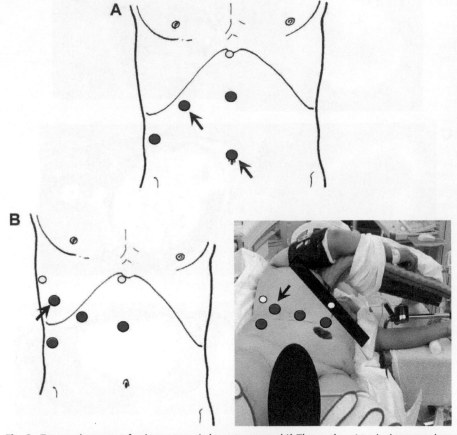

Fig. 2. Trocar placement for laparoscopic hepatectomy. (*A*) The authors' typical trocar placement for laparoscopic hepatectomy on the right liver. During fluorescence imaging, a laparoscope can be inserted from the umbilicus trocar or the subcostal trocar (*arrows*), depending on the tumor location. In laparoscopic hepatectomy for the tumor located in segment 7 and/or 8, 1 or 2 balloon-tipped trocars are deployed from the intercostal space through the diaphragm (intercostal trocars; *B*). A laparoscope is usually inserted from the intercostal trocar (*arrow*) for fluorescence imaging on the subphrenic hepatic surfaces.

fluorescence imaging, it is important to insert the laparoscope through the subcostal or intercostal trocars and to orient its tip vertically to the hepatic surfaces to efficiently obtain the fluorescence signal.[7,8]

Fluorescence Imaging Systems

When we applied fluorescence imaging to laparoscopic cholecystectomy and hepatectomy in the late 2000s for the first time,[11,12] only a prototype laparoscopic imaging system with a standard-definition image quality was available. Since then, several laparoscopic near-infrared imaging systems from almost all major medical device companies are available. The improved image quality and usability provides favorable working conditions for surgeons. Nevertheless, care should be taken to recognize differences in the visualizability of fluorescence images and quality of color images among the imaging system used.[7] Especially in the planning and evaluation of clinical studies on fluorescence imaging, the differences between the various products need to be taken into account and can be seen in the figures presented in this article.

Surgical Procedure

Liver cancer identification

The technique of ICG fluorescent imaging of liver cancer is straightforward: once ICG (0.5 mg/kg) is administered within 2 weeks before surgery, fluorescent images of liver cancers can be obtained intraoperatively by simply placing the tip of a near-infrared laparoscopic imaging system close to the liver surface.[3,8] Fluorescence imaging can be used at any time, not only at the level of the hepatic surfaces, but also deeper in the liver parenchyma as the transection planes are being developed. This process can be helpful for surgeons to confirm appropriate surgical margins during the hepatic parenchymal transection (**Fig. 3**).[8]

Because ICG fluorescence imaging of liver cancer is not based on a cancer-specific interaction between ICG and the cancer, but simply on a reduced ability of cancer and noncancerous tissue surrounding the actual cancer to secret bile (and thereby ICG), a false-positive rate of the current technique is high (around 40%).[3,6] Therefore, if small previously unknown lesions are detected by intraoperative fluorescence imaging, the authors consider additional resection only when malignancy is also suggested by other modalities, such as palpation and/or ultrasound imaging.

Fluorescence cholangiography

As mentioned, to obtain clear fluorescence images of the bile ducts, ICG (2.5 mg or 0.5 mg/kg for liver function test) is optimally administered intravenously before surgery. For the intraoperative intravenous injection of ICG for fluorescence cholangiography, ICG should be administered at least 15 minutes before the fluorescence imaging so that the background fluorescence signal is decreased.[7,13] For the visualization of microscopic extension of bile duct cancer fluorescent cholangiography provides useful information on the extrahepatic bile duct anatomy. Nevertheless, the microscopic extend of the cancer along the bile duct cannot be visualized. Detailed information on bile duct anatomy may enhance the safety of complicated laparoscopic hepatobiliary surgery for cancers in proximity of major bile ducts (**Fig. 4**).[8]

Delineation of hepatic segments

Two fluorescence imaging approaches for the identification of hepatic segmental boundaries are available today: positive and negative staining techniques.[14] For the positive staining technique, the portal branch to be stained is punctured under

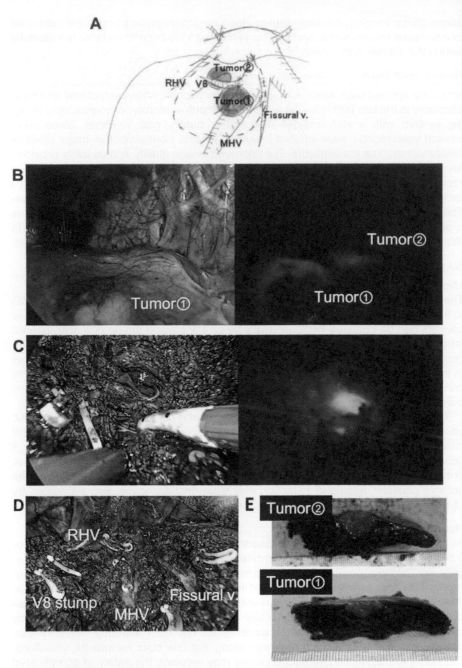

Fig. 3. Identification of liver cancer by indocyanine green (ICG) fluorescence imaging during laparoscopic hepatectomy. A wedge resection of hepatic segment 4/8 is indicated to remove 2 colorectal liver metastases, dividing a drainage vein of segment 8 (V8) and preserving the middle hepatic vein (MHV) and the right hepatic vein (RHV; *A*). The tumors are identified on the hepatic surfaces before parenchymal transection by fluorescence imaging (*right*) as well as white-light color imaging (*left*; *B*). Fluorescence imaging can be used repeatedly on the hepatic raw surfaces during parenchymal transection, enabling identification of the tumor

ultrasound guidance and 5 to 10 mL of diluted ICG solution (0.05–0.25 mg/mL) is directly injected. Subsequently, ICG is taken up by hepatocytes of the corresponding hepatic segments, leading to long-lasting visualization of the segment by fluorescence imaging during the hepatectomy. Although the positive staining technique using blue dye (indigo carmine)[15] has been used as a standard surgical technique for the identification of segmental boundaries in open hepatectomy for more than 30 years, reproducing this technique in laparoscopic surgery is technically demanding compared with the negative staining technique described elsewhere in this article.

For the negative staining technique, a portal pedicle corresponding with the tumor-bearing hepatic segment is occluded with a vascular clamp, followed by intravenous injection of ICG (1.25–2.50 mg). Then, fluorescence imaging delineates the boundaries between ischemic hepatic segments to be removed and the nonischemic liver. This ICG-based delineation is more obvious than ischemic demarcation under white light imaging (regular laparoscopic images) only.[8] The major advantage in the use of ICG fluorescence imaging during hepatic resection is that it enables identification of segmental boundaries not only on the hepatic surfaces before hepatectomy, but also on the exposed surfaces during the parenchymal dissection (**Fig. 5**). In contrast, hepatic segments stained in blue by the conventional technique become unidentifiable within 2 to 3 minutes after the injection of indigo carmine because it washes out from the liver and is renally excreted.

Fluorescence angiography and perfusion assessment

Fluorescence imaging by intraoperative intravenous injection of ICG can also be used for the visualization of the arterial/venous anatomy and assessment of blood perfusion. For this technique, a bolus injection of ICG (2.5 mg) through ideally a central venous catheter is the optimal approach to obtain a high fluorescence signal in the vessels (**Fig. 6**). According to the authors' experience, the present technique has the potential to determine the need for vessel reconstruction. It also allows to evaluate blood perfusion through an anastomosis.

PUBLISHED REPORTS

Since the first report of fluorescence cholangiography using intravenous injection of ICG during laparoscopic cholecystectomy in 2009,[11] up to 1000 clinical cases of minimally invasive cholecystectomy with the use of fluorescence cholangiography have been reported.[7,13,16–35] In these series, sufficient bile duct detectability ranging from 70% to 100% have been reported (**Table 1**). Previous systemic reviews have described the potential advantages of fluorescence cholangiography over conventional radiographic imaging in the real-time visualization of the extrahepatic bile duct anatomy during laparoscopic cholecystectomy.[35] Recently, multicenter prospective trials have been conducted worldwide to confirm the efficacy of fluorescence cholangiography as a routine surgical procedure during cholecystectomy.[36] Other applications of fluorescence cholangiography include the identification of bile ducts

located close to the future dissection planes, through visualization of ICG fluorescence signals emitted from noncancerous hepatic parenchyma surrounding the tumor. This information is useful for surgeons to change hepatic transection planes more deeply to avoid tumor exposure (C). (D, E) Hepatic raw surfaces after the resection and cut surfaces of the resected specimens, respectively.

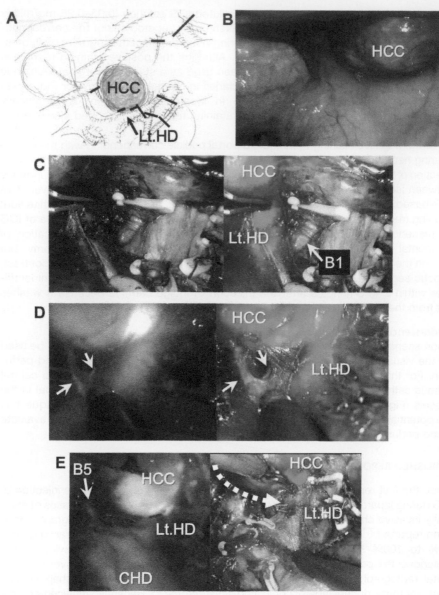

Fig. 4. Laparoscopic left hepatectomy using fluorescence cholangiography. Laparoscopic left hepatectomy preserving the Spiegel lobe is scheduled to treat hepatocellular carcinoma (HCC) located in hepatic segment 4 and attaching to the left hepatic duct (Lt. HD; *A* and *B*). In this patient, fluorescence cholangiography can be performed by using the indocyanine green (ICG) that was injected intravenously at a dose of 0.5 mg/kg on the day before the surgery for preoperative liver function estimation. After division of the left hepatic artery, fluorescence cholangiography identifies a branch of hepatic duct draining the Spiegel lobe to be preserved (B1; *C*). During detachment of HCC from the Lt. HD, fluorescence cholangiography visualizes 2 thin branches of hepatic duct directly draining into the Lt. HD (*arrows*), which is a potential risk of bile duct injury and postoperative bile leak (*D*). Fluorescence imaging is used again to determine a hepatic transection line (*dotted arrow*) toward the Lt. HD, preserving the hepatic duct draining segment 5 (B5; *E*). After completion

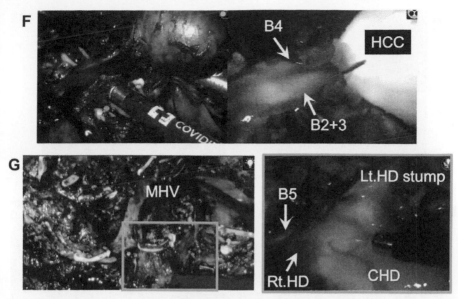

Fig. 4. (*continued*).

during hepatectomy,[8,37] the Kasai procedure for biliary atresia,[38] and deroofing of hepatic cysts.[39]

The first clinical series of intraoperative fluorescence imaging using ICG for identification of liver cancer was also reported in 2009.[3,40] Since then, more than 20 clinical studies have evaluated the efficacy of ICG fluorescence imaging for the identification of primary and secondary hepatic tumors.[4,8,41–50] Potential advantages of the present technique lie in its feasibility and high sensitivity. In fact, a retrospective comparative study revealed that the use of ICG fluorescence imaging was associated with the identification of more and smaller tumors. Despite these early findings, the impact of this technique on long-term outcomes needs to be evaluated further in prospective studies.[51] Further, novel fluorophores specific to adenocarcinoma tissues have been developed. In the near future, these new intraoperative imaging techniques may enable the visualization of the actual cancer, which may help surgeons to optimize the extent of resection during hepatobiliary surgery, including pancreatectomy.

Anatomic hepatectomy has been performed for more than 30 years as a safe and potentially curative and surgical procedure for the treatment of liver cancer. Hepatocellular carcinoma has a tendency to spread along the portal venous system. In this context, anatomic segmentectomy may be associated with a lower risk of postoperative recurrence than nonanatomic limited resection.[52] In the original description of

---

of hepatic transection and division of the left hepatic vein, the Lt. HD is encircled. Fluorescence imaging visualizes the confluence of the hepatic ducts draining segment 4 (B4) and left lateral section (B2+3; F). (G) The hepatic raw surfaces after left hepatectomy preserving the middle hepatic vein (MHV). Fluorescence cholangiography suggests that the left hepatic duct is accurately closed without any bile leaks or injuries on the right hepatic duct (Rt. HD). CHD, common hepatic duct.

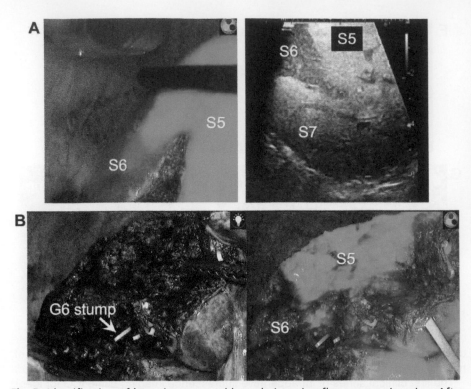

Fig. 5. Identification of hepatic segmental boundaries using fluorescence imaging. After the closure of Glissonian sheath of segment 6 (G6), indocyanine green (ICG; 2.5 mg) and ultrasound contrast agent are injected intravenously. Then, the boundaries of ischemic segment 6 regions (S6) between segment 5 (S5) and segment 7 (S7) without ischemia are clearly delineated by fluorescence imaging (*left*) and contrast-enhanced ultrasound imaging (*right*; *A*). The segmental boundaries can be identified not only from the subphrenic hepatic surfaces, but also on the hepatic raw surfaces during parenchymal dissection (*B*).

this technique by Makuuchi and colleagues,[15] boundaries of hepatic segments were identified by injection of indigo carmine solution into the segmental branch of the portal vein under ultrasound guidance. Subsequently the hepatic surface of the corresponding segments stained blue. However, the staining usually disappears within minutes after the injection of indigo-carmine. In 2008, Aoki and colleagues[17] first applied fluorescence imaging to intraoperative hepatic segmentation using ICG in place of indigo carmine. In 2012, the authors applied ICG fluorescence imaging to hepatic segmentation during laparoscopic hepatectomy.[14] The authors reported reducing the dose of ICG to be injected into the portal branch, which enabled long-lasting visualization of segmental boundaries while minimizing background fluorescence signal in the surrounding liver.[53] The commercial introduction of the fluorescence imaging systems that enable superimposition of fluorescence signals on white light images facilitates the identification of hepatic segments by ICG fluorescence imaging. This technique may become a standard during open as well as laparoscopic hepatectomy in the future.[8,54]

Although few articles have been published on the use of ICG fluorescence imaging for perfusion assessment during hepatobiliary and pancreatic surgery, this technique

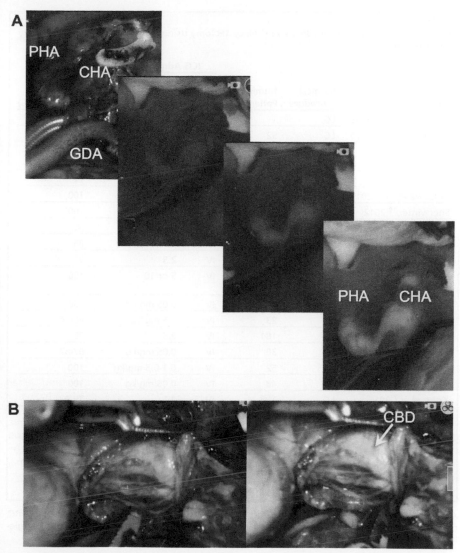

Fig. 6. Fluorescence angiography and cholangiography during laparoscopic pancreatoduodenectomy. During laparoscopic pancreatoduodenectomy, fluorescence angiography is performed to confirm hepatic arterial flow via the common hepatic artery (CHA) and the proper hepatic artery (PHA) by injecting indocyanine green (ICG; 2.5 mg) intravenously after closure of the gastroduodenal artery (GDA; A). After the administration of ICG for angiography, fluorescence cholangiography can also be used to discriminate the common bile duct (CBD) from the lymphatic ducts and small vessels in the hepatoduodenal ligament (B).

may develop into an essential intraoperative diagnostic tool for the prediction and prevention of ischemia, organ failure,[55] digestive tract perforation, or anastomotic leakage.[56] To enhance the efficacy and reproducibility of perfusion assessment by fluorescence imaging, a reliable method for quantitative and real-time measurement of fluorescence signals after injection of ICG needs to be further developed in the future.

Table 1
Previous reports of minimally invasive cholecystectomy using fluorescence cholangiography (2008–2016)

Reference	Surgical Procedure	Number of Patients	ICG Administration Route	Dose (mg)	Bile Duct Detectability Before/After Dissection (%)
Ishizawa et al,[11] 2009	LC	1	IV	2.5	100/100
Ishizawa et al,[13] 2010	LC	52	IV	2.5	96/100
Tagaya,[16] 2010	OC	4	IV	2.5	100
	LC	8			100
Aoki et al,[17] 2010	LC	14	IV	12.5	71
Ishizawa et al,[18] 2011	SILC	7	IV	2.5	100
Sherwinter,[19] 2012	LC	1	IV	1 mL	100
Buchs et al,[20] 2013	SIRC	23	IV	2.5	ND
Spinoglio et al,[21] 2013	SIRC	45	IV	2.5	98
Schols et al,[22] 2013	LC	30	IV	2.5	97
Verbeek et al,[23] 2014	OC	27	IV	5 or 10	100
	LC	14			
Larsen et al,[24] 2014	LC	35	IV	0.05 mg/kg	100
Prevot et al,[25] 2014	LC	23	IV	0.5 mg/kg	48/74
Daskalaki et al,[26] 2014	RC	184	IV	2.5	98
van Dam et al,[27] 2015	LC	30	IV	0.05 mg/kg	67/87
Boni et al,[28] 2015	LC	52	IV	0.1-0.5 mg/kg	100
Dip et al,[29] 2015	LC	43	IV	0.05 mg/kg	100
Kono et al,[7] 2015	LC	108	IV	2.5	79/92
Osayi et al,[30] 2015	LC	82	IV	2.5	95
Igami et al,[31] 2016	SILC	21	IV	2.5	71
Dip et al,[32] 2016	LC (obese)	71	IV	0.05 mg/kg	70
Zarrinpar et al,[33] 2016	LC	37	IV	0.02, 0.04, 0.08, and 0.25 mg/kg	ND
Tsutsui et al,[34] 2016	LC	1	IV	25	100

Abbreviations: LC, laparoscopic cholecystectomy; ND, no data; OC, open cholecystectomy; RC, robot-assisted cholecystectomy; SILC, single-incision laparoscopic cholecystectomy; SIRC, single-incision robot-assisted cholecystectomy.

SUMMARY

Applications of fluorescence imaging using ICG during hepatobiliary and pancreatic surgery include (i) liver cancer identification, (ii) fluorescence cholangiography, (iii) hepatic segments delineation, (iv) fluorescence angiography, and (v) perfusion assessment. With the development of target-specific fluorophores and imaging technology, intraoperative fluorescence imaging will become an essential intraoperative navigation tool, enhancing both accuracy and safety of minimally invasive surgery.

REFERENCES

1. Dip FD, Ishizawa T, Kokudo N, et al, editors. Fluorescence imaging for surgeons. Springer International Publishing Switzerland; 2015.

2. Landsman ML, Kwant G, Mook GA, et al. Light-absorbing properties, stability, and spectral stabilization of indocyanine green. J Appl Physiol 1976;40:575–83.
3. Ishizawa T, Fukushima N, Shibahara J, et al. Real-time identification of liver cancers by using indocyanine green fluorescent imaging. Cancer 2009;115: 2491–504.
4. van der Vorst JR, Schaafsma BE, Hutteman M, et al. Near-infrared fluorescence-guided resection of colorectal liver metastases. Cancer 2013;119:3411–8.
5. Ishizawa T, Harada N, Muraoka A, et al. Scientific basis and clinical application of ICG fluorescence imaging: hepatobiliary cancer. Open Surg Oncol J 2010;2: 31–6.
6. Ishizawa T, Masuda K, Urano Y, et al. Mechanistic background and clinical applications of indocyanine green-fluorescence imaging of hepatocellular carcinoma. Ann Surg Oncol 2014;21:440–8.
7. Kono Y, Ishizawa T, Tani K, et al. Techniques of fluorescence cholangiography during laparoscopic cholecystectomy for better delineation of the bile duct anatomy. Medicine (Baltimore) 2015;94:e1005.
8. Terasawa M, Ishizawa T, Saiura A, et al. Applications of fusion fluorescence imaging using indocyanine green in laparoscopic hepatectomy. Surg Endosc 2017; 31:5111–8.
9. Ishizawa T, Gumbs AA, Kokudo N, et al. Laparoscopic segmentectomy of the liver: from segment I to VIII. Ann Surg 2012;256:959–64.
10. Ichida H, Ishizawa T, Saiura A, et al. Use of intercostal trocars for laparoscopic resection of subphrenic hepatic tumors. Surg Endosc 2017;31:1280–6.
11. Ishizawa T, Bandai Y, Kokudo N. Fluorescent cholangiography using indocyanine green for laparoscopic cholecystectomy: an initial experience. Arch Surg 2009; 144:381–2.
12. Ishizawa T, Bandai Y, Kokudo N, et al. Indocyanine green-fluorescent imaging of hepatocellular carcinoma during laparoscopic hepatectomy: an initial experience. Asian J Endosc Surg 2010;3:42–5.
13. Ishizawa T, Bandai Y, Ijichi M, et al. Fluorescent cholangiography illuminating the biliary tree during laparoscopic cholecystectomy. Br J Surg 2010;97:1369–77.
14. Ishizawa T, Zuker NB, Kokudo N, et al. Positive and negative staining of hepatic segments by use of fluorescent imaging techniques during laparoscopic hepatectomy. Arch Surg 2012;147:393–4.
15. Makuuchi M, Hasegawa H, Yamazaki S. Ultrasonically guided subsegmentectomy. Surg Gynecol Obstet 1985;161:346–50.
16. Tagaya N, Shimoda M, Kato M, et al. Intraoperative exploration of biliary anatomy using fluorescence imaging of indocyanine green in experimental and clinical cholecystectomies. J Hepatobiliary Pancreat Sci 2010;17:595–600.
17. Aoki T, Murakami M, Yasuda D, et al. Intraoperative fluorescent imaging using indocyanine green for liver mapping and cholangiography. J Hepatobiliary Pancreat Sci 2010;17:590–4.
18. Ishizawa T, Kaneko J, Inoue Y, et al. Application of fluorescent cholangiography to single-incision laparoscopic cholecystectomy. Surg Endosc 2011;25:2631–6.
19. Sherwinter DA. Identification of anomalous biliary anatomy using near-infrared cholangiography. J Gastrointest Surg 2012;16:1814–5.
20. Buchs NC, Pugin F, Azagury DE, et al. Real-time near-infrared fluorescent cholangiography could shorten operative time during robotic single-site cholecystectomy. Surg Endosc 2013;27:3897–901.

21. Spinoglio G, Priora F, Bianchi PP, et al. Real-time near-infrared (NIR) fluorescent cholangiography in single-site robotic cholecystectomy (SSRC): a single-institutional prospective study. Surg Endosc 2013;27:2156–62.

22. Schols RM, Bouvy ND, van Dam RM, et al. Combined vascular and biliary fluorescence imaging in laparoscopic cholecystectomy. Surg Endosc 2013;27:4511–7.

23. Verbeek FP, Schaafsma BE, Tummers QR, et al. Optimization of near-infrared fluorescence cholangiography for open and laparoscopic surgery. Surg Endosc 2014;28:1076–82.

24. Larsen SS, Schulze S, Bisgaard T. Non-radiographic intraoperative fluorescent cholangiography is feasible. Dan Med J 2014;61:A4891.

25. Prevot F, Rebibo L, Cosse C, et al. Effectiveness of intraoperative cholangiography using indocyanine green (versus contrast fluid) for the correct assessment of extrahepatic bile ducts during day-case laparoscopic cholecystectomy. J Gastrointest Surg 2014;18:1462–8.

26. Daskalaki D, Fernandes E, Wang X, et al. Indocyanine green (ICG) fluorescent cholangiography during robotic cholecystectomy: results of 184 consecutive cases in a single institution. Surg Innov 2014;21:615–21.

27. van Dam DA, Ankersmit M, van de Ven P, et al. Comparing near-infrared imaging with indocyanine green to conventional imaging during laparoscopic cholecystectomy: a prospective crossover study. J Laparoendosc Adv Surg Tech A 2015;25:486–92.

28. Boni L, David G, Mangano A, et al. Clinical applications of indocyanine green (ICG) enhanced fluorescence in laparoscopic surgery. Surg Endosc 2015;29:2046–55.

29. Dip F, Roy M, Menzo EL, et al. Routine use of fluorescent incisionless cholangiography as a new imaging modality during laparoscopic cholecystectomy. Surg Endosc 2015;29:1621–6.

30. Osayi SN, Wendling MR, Drosdeck JM, et al. Near-infrared fluorescent cholangiography facilitates identification of biliary anatomy during laparoscopic cholecystectomy. Surg Endosc 2015;29:368–75.

31. Igami T, Nojiri M, Shinohara K, et al. Clinical value and pitfalls of fluorescent cholangiography during single-incision laparoscopic cholecystectomy. Surg Today 2016;46:1443–50.

32. Dip F, Nguyen D, Montorfano L, et al. Accuracy of near infrared-guided surgery in morbidly obese subjects undergoing laparoscopic cholecystectomy. Obes Surg 2015;26:525–30.

33. Zarrinpar A, Dutson EP, Mobley C, et al. Intraoperative laparoscopic near-infrared fluorescence cholangiography to facilitate anatomical identification: when to give indocyanine green and how much. Surg Innov 2016;23:360–5.

34. Tsutsui N, Yoshida M, Kitajima M, et al. Laparoscopic cholecystectomy using the PINPOINT endoscopic fluorescence imaging system with intraoperative fluorescent imaging: a case report. Int J Surg Case Rep 2016;21:129–32.

35. Vlek SL, van Dam DA, Rubinstein SM, et al. Biliary tract visualization using near-infrared imaging with indocyanine green during laparoscopic cholecystectomy: results of a systematic review. Surg Endosc 2017;31:2731–42.

36. van den Bos J, Schols RM, Luyer MD, et al. Near-infrared fluorescence cholangiography assisted laparoscopic cholecystectomy versus conventional laparoscopic cholecystectomy (FALCON trial): study protocol for a multicentre randomised controlled trial. BMJ Open 2016;6:e011668.

07. Hong SK, Lee KW, Kim HS, et al. Optimal bile duct division using real-time indocyanine green near-infrared fluorescence cholangiography during laparoscopic donor hepatectomy. Liver Transpl 2017;23:847–52.
38. Hirayama Y, Iinuma Y, Yokoyama N, et al. Near-infrared fluorescence cholangiography with indocyanine green for biliary atresia. Real-time imaging during the Kasai procedure: a pilot study. Pediatr Surg Int 2015;31:1177–82.
39. Tanaka M, Inoue Y, Mise Y, et al. Laparoscopic deroofing for polycystic liver disease using laparoscopic fusion indocyanine green fluorescence imaging. Surg Endosc 2016;30:2620–3.
40. Gotoh K, Yamada T, Ishikawa O, et al. A novel image-guided surgery of hepatocellular carcinoma by indocyanine green fluorescence imaging navigation. J Surg Oncol 2009;100:75–9.
41. Uchiyama K, Ueno M, Ozawa S, et al. Combined use of contrast-enhanced intraoperative ultrasonography and a fluorescence navigation system for identifying hepatic metastases. World J Surg 2010;34:2953–9.
42. Yokoyama N, Otani T, Hashidate H, et al. Real-time detection of hepatic micrometastases from pancreatic cancer by intraoperative fluorescence imaging: preliminary results of a prospective study. Cancer 2012;118:2813–9.
43. Morita Y, Sakaguchi T, Unno N, et al. Detection of hepatocellular carcinomas with near-infrared fluorescence imaging using indocyanine green: its usefulness and limitation. Int J Clin Oncol 2013;18:232–41.
44. Ishizuka M, Kubota K, Kita J, et al. Intraoperative observation using a fluorescence imaging instrument during hepatic resection for liver metastasis from colorectal cancer. Hepatogastroenterology 2012;59:90–2.
45. Peloso A, Franchi E, Canepa MC, et al. Combined use of intraoperative ultrasound and indocyanine green fluorescence imaging to detect liver metastases from colorectal cancer. HPB (Oxford) 2013;15:928–34.
46. Kudo H, Ishizawa T, Tani K, et al. Visualization of subcapsular hepatic malignancy by indocyanine-green fluorescence imaging during laparoscopic hepatectomy. Surg Endosc 2014;28:2504–8.
47. Abo T, Nanashima A, Tobinaga S, et al. Usefulness of intraoperative diagnosis of hepatic tumors located at the liver surface and hepatic segmental visualization using indocyanine green-photodynamic eye imaging. Eur J Surg Oncol 2015; 41:257–64.
48. Shimada S, Ohtsubo S, Ogasawara K, et al. Macro- and microscopic findings of ICG fluorescence in liver tumors. World J Surg Oncol 2015;13:198.
49. Kawaguchi Y, Nagai M, Nomura Y, et al. Usefulness of indocyanine green-fluorescence imaging during laparoscopic hepatectomy to visualize subcapsular hard-to-identify hepatic malignancy. J Surg Oncol 2015;112:514–6.
50. Tummers QR, Verbeek FP, Prevoo HA, et al. First experience on laparoscopic near-infrared fluorescence imaging of hepatic uveal melanoma metastases using indocyanine green. Surg innovation 2015;22:20–5.
51. Handgraaf HJM, Boogerd LSF, Hoppener DJ, et al. Long-term follow-up after near-infrared fluorescence-guided resection of colorectal liver metastases: a retrospective multicenter analysis. Eur J Surg Oncol 2017;43:1463–71.
52. Hasegawa K, Kokudo N, Imamura H, et al. Prognostic impact of anatomic resection for hepatocellular carcinoma. Ann Surg 2005;242:252–9.
53. Inoue Y, Arita J, Sakamoto T, et al. Anatomical liver resections guided by 3-dimensional parenchymal staining using fusion indocyanine green fluorescence imaging. Ann Surg 2015;262:105–11.

54. Miyata A, Ishizawa T, Tani K, et al. Reappraisal of a dye-staining technique for anatomic hepatectomy by the concomitant use of indocyanine green-fluorescence imaging. J Am Coll Surg 2015;221:e27–36.
55. Kawaguchi Y, Ishizawa T, Miyata Y, et al. Portal uptake function in veno-occlusive regions evaluated by real-time fluorescent imaging using indocyanine green. J Hepatol 2013;58:247–53.
56. Jafari MD, Wexner SD, Martz JE, et al. Perfusion assessment in laparoscopic left-sided/anterior resection (PILLAR II): a multi-institutional study. J Am Coll Surg 2015;220:82–92.

Minimally Invasive Staging Surgery for Cancer

Noah A. Cohen, MD, Thomas Peter Kingham, MD*

KEYWORDS

- Staging • Laparoscopy • Cancer • Gastric • Pancreas • Colorectal liver metastasis

KEY POINTS

- Staging laparoscopy (SL) is a minimally invasive modality used to assess for radiographically occult metastatic disease and local resectability in selected patients with gastrointestinal malignancies.
- SL may avoid nontherapeutic laparotomy in patients with unresectable cancer.
- SL is associated with shorter length of hospital stay and time to receipt of systemic therapy when compared with nontherapeutic laparotomy.
- Patients with distal gastroesophageal junction cancer and locally advanced gastric cancer should have SL with peritoneal washings for cytology before planned resection.
- SL should be considered for selected patients with hepatopancreatobiliary malignancies before planned resection.

INTRODUCTION TO STAGING LAPAROSCOPY

Staging laparoscopy (SL) is a diagnostic modality used in selected patients with gastrointestinal malignancies to assess for radiographically occult metastatic disease and tumor resectability. The use of SL may avoid nontherapeutic laparotomy in patients with unresectable tumors. Compared with nontherapeutic laparotomy, SL is associated with decreased postoperative pain, length of stay (LOS), and time to receiving systemic therapy in patients with unresectable cancer.[1–4] Detection of metastatic and locally unresectable disease has improved with advances in preoperative imaging, such as multidetector computed tomography (CT), magnetic resonance cholangiopancreatography (MRCP), and endoscopic ultrasound (EUS), and the application of SL has become more selective.[5–9]

Staging Laparoscopy Yield and Accuracy

SL yield is defined as the number of patients with unresectable disease identified during SL divided by the total number of patients who undergo SL. Accuracy is defined as

Disclosure Statement: The authors have nothing to disclose
Department of Surgery, Memorial Sloan Kettering Cancer Center, 1275 York Avenue, New York, NY 10065, USA
* Corresponding author.
E-mail address: kinghamt@mskcc.org

Surg Oncol Clin N Am 28 (2019) 61–77
https://doi.org/10.1016/j.soc.2018.07.006
surgonc.theclinics.com
1055-3207/19/© 2018 Elsevier Inc. All rights reserved.

the number of patients with unresectable disease identified during SL divided by the total number of patients with unresectable disease.

SURGICAL TECHNIQUE
One-Stage Versus Two-Stage Staging Laparoscopy

SL is performed under general anesthesia, either before a planned definitive resection during a single anesthetic event (1 stage) or as a separate procedure (2 stage). The benefits of 2-stage SL include the ability to obtain final pathologic evaluation of peritoneal washings and biopsy specimens, and to better manage valuable operating room time, as allocated time for a planned resection will not be wasted if unresectable disease is discovered during SL. Conversely, a 2-stage SL will subject patients to an additional general anesthesia event and its attendant risks.

Technique

The patient is placed supine, and general anesthesia is induced. A supraumbilical port is placed under direct vision, and the abdomen is insufflated with carbon dioxide to 15 mm Hg. Additional ports are placed under direct vision. The abdomen is explored using an angled laparoscope, and all peritoneal surfaces, the paracolic gutters, the pelvis, and the liver are inspected for metastatic disease.

For patients with gastric cancer (GC) or gastroesophageal junction (GEJ) tumors, 2-stage SL is most common, and the porta hepatis, celiac axis, and the lesser and greater curves of the stomach are inspected; abnormal lymph nodes are sampled. The anterior surface of the stomach is examined for gross tumor extension through the serosa and local invasion. For a posteriorly located tumor, the lesser sac is opened, and the posterior aspect of the stomach is examined.

SL for hepatopancreatobiliary (HPB) malignancies is performed in a similar manner, typically as a 1-stage procedure. All peritoneal surfaces, including the anterior and posterior surfaces of the liver, the porta hepatis, the gastrohepatic omentum, the duodenum, the transverse mesocolon, the ligament of Treitz, and the celiac region, are examined. In the absence of gross metastatic disease, laparoscopic ultrasound (US) is performed, which may identify additional disease in 10% of patients, including deep liver metastases and abnormal lymph nodes.[10] Laparoscopic US may also be used to assess the relationship of the tumor with major vascular and biliary structures to determine local resectability.[11] Minimizing cautery when sampling suspicious lesions is recommended.

SL yield and accuracy may be affected by intraoperative technique because peritoneal and surface liver metastases may be identified by SL, whereas nodal metastasis and vascular invasion are more challenging to determine laparoscopically.[12,13] Laparoscopic surface inspection without mobilization of structures, lymph node sampling, or laparoscopic US may result in a lower yield and accuracy compared with more extensive exploration.[12,14]

Cytology

If present, ascites fluid is aspirated for cytology. For patients with GC or GEJ cancer without ascites or macroscopic metastatic disease, peritoneal washings are obtained for cytology to assess for microscopic peritoneal disease.[15] The patient is placed in the Trendelenburg position, and 200 mL saline is instilled into the left and right upper quadrants, which is then aspirated and collected for cytology. The patient is then placed in the reverse Trendelenburg position and 200 mL saline is instilled into the pelvis and aspirated and collected for cytology. Saline aspirates are centrifuged, and cells are fixed, mounted on slides, and stained using the Papanicolaou technique.[16]

Risks of Staging Laparoscopy

SL is safe, with low morbidity and minimal mortality. Morbidity is related to bleeding, infection, and bowel injury from port placement or adhesiolysis.[17–19] Patients must be able to tolerate pneumoperitoneum and be medically fit for general anesthesia.

Port-Site Metastasis

Despite early reports of port site metastasis after laparoscopic oncologic surgery, contemporary series report a <1% port site recurrence rate.[20–23] Various factors, such a carbon dioxide insufflation, wound contamination with tumor cells during tumor extraction or laparoscopic instrument exchange, and immune changes after laparoscopy, have all been implicated.[23] However, port site metastasis typically occurs with local and distant recurrence,[21] and port site and laparotomy incision recurrence occur at a similar rate,[22] suggesting that port site recurrence be considered a marker of disease biology rather than a technical complication of minimal access surgery.

STAGING LAPAROSCOPY FOR GASTROESOPHAGEAL JUNCTION AND GASTRIC CANCER
Indications

Combined with cross-sectional imaging and EUS, SL with peritoneal cytology is a critical diagnostic component for patients with distal GEJ tumors and clinical T3/T4 GC, before definitive resection or initiation of neoadjuvant chemotherapy, or when multivisceral resection is anticipated due to a locally invasive tumor.[24–29]

Contraindications

Patients with tumors causing bleeding, obstruction, or perforation who require palliative procedures should not undergo SL.[7] Patients with clinical T1/T2 tumors by EUS have a low risk of peritoneal metastasis and do not benefit from SL.[7,30,31] Dense adhesions from prior upper abdominal operations may limit safe laparoscopic exploration.

Accuracy and Alteration of Management in Gastroesophageal Junction and Gastric Cancer

SL may alter management in up to half of patients with clinical T3/T4 GC.[32,33] In a study of 657 patients with GC or GEJ cancer at Memorial Sloan Kettering Cancer Center (MSKCC) between 1993 and 2002, radiographically occult metastatic disease was discovered during SL in 208 (31%) patients, most commonly in the peritoneum (72%), liver (8%), and para-aortic lymph nodes (8%).[7] Tumor location (GEJ or whole stomach) and lymphadenopathy on CT independently predicted detection of M1 disease. Similar findings were reported in a study from England including 416 patients with radiographically localized GC or esophageal cancer from 1997 to 2003.[26] A meta-analysis concluded that SL was most accurate for M staging, compared with T and N staging, with an overall accuracy of 85% to 98.9%, sensitivity of 64.3% to 94%, and specificity of 80% to 100%.[33] Nontherapeutic laparotomy was avoided in 8.5% to 43.8% of cases, and treatment was altered in 8.5% to 59.6% of cases. When only patients with T3/T4 tumors were analyzed, SL changed management in 25% to 54% of patients. A Surveillance, Epidemiology, and End Results database analysis showed that 151 of 506 (29.8%) GC patients who underwent SL did not have a subsequent surgical procedure.[34] Those patients who only underwent SL had a shorter hospital LOS and lower in-hospital mortality compared with patients who underwent nontherapeutic laparotomy.

Peritoneal Cytology

The most common mode of metastasis in GC is the shedding of tumor cells directly into the peritoneal cavity, which is classified as stage IV disease.[35–37] Approximately 40% of patients with stage III GC have positive cytology.[38,39] Compared with conventional cytology, reverse-transcriptase polymerase chain reaction for carcinoembryonic antigen is more sensitive for detection of free cancer cells collected from peritoneal washings.[40,41] Patients with advanced T-stage tumors are more likely to have positive peritoneal cytology, which is classified as M1 disease in American Joint Committee on Cancer 8th Edition Cancer Staging Manual[42] and is associated with worse outcomes. A Japanese study including 1297 patients found that 4% had positive cytology, which was more common in patients with higher T stage (T3/T4 vs T2) and poorly differentiated tumors.[43] Patients with positive cytology had worse 5-year overall survival, 2% versus 58% (P<.001). Similarly, a Brazilian study of 222 patients found that patients with positive cytology had a 10.5-months mean survival compared with 61 months in cytology-negative patients (P = .00001).[44] A study of 127 patients from MSKCC reported that none of the patients with T1/T2 tumors had positive cytology, whereas 3 of 31 patients with T3/T4 tumors had positive cytology.[30] Those patients with positive cytology had worse survival despite attempted resection for cure, equivalent to patients with macroscopic peritoneal disease. Similarly, a study from Belfast reported equivalent median survival in patients with macroscopic and microscopic peritoneal disease (208 days vs 368 days, P = .219).[19] In another study from MSKCC including 371 patients with radiographically localized GC who underwent SL with peritoneal cytology followed by R0 resection, median survival was significantly worse in the 24 (6.5%) patients with positive peritoneal cytology, 14.8 months, compared with 98.5 months in cytology-negative patients (P<.0001).[45] Multivariate analysis identified preoperative T and N stage, tumor location, and positive cytology as significant independent preoperative predictors of survival, with positive cytology the most significant factor. Another Japanese study including 701 patients reported worse survival in patients with macroscopic or microscopic peritoneal disease compared with patients with localized disease, with a 7.8% 5-year survival in patients with positive peritoneal cytology.[46] Similar findings were observed in a Korean study.[16]

Staging Laparoscopy and Neoadjuvant Therapy

SL should be performed before initiation of neoadjuvant chemotherapy, which is recommended for patients with T3 or greater GC.[32] Repeat SL after completion of chemotherapy may identify patients with progressive disease to avoid nontherapeutic laparotomy and may identify patients with positive peritoneal cytology who convert to cytology-negative, which may inform prognosis. Following a negative SL and completing neoadjuvant chemotherapy, 136 patients underwent repeat SL and 80 patients proceeded directly to laparotomy at MSKCC.[47] Radiographically occult metastatic disease was identified in approximately 7% of patients in both groups, and outcomes in these patients, independent of resection, were worse than those without evidence of metastatic disease. A study from MSKCC reported that 27 of 48 GC patients with positive peritoneal cytology on initial SL converted to cytology-negative on repeat SL after receiving systemic chemotherapy.[48] Those patients had improved survival compared with persistently cytology-positive patients, median disease-specific survival 2.5 years versus 1.4 years (P = .0003). Similarly, a German study of T3/T4 GC patients with positive cytology reported improved survival in patients who converted to cytology-negative after systemic chemotherapy.[49]

Summary: Staging Laparoscopy in Gastric and Gastroesophageal Cancer

SL is essential in the management of T3/T4 GC and GEJ adenocarcinoma in patients who do not otherwise require a palliative gastrectomy. Despite the improvement of preoperative imaging, SL and peritoneal cytology identifies 40% of patients with unresectable disease, which may avoid a nontherapeutic laparotomy.

STAGING LAPAROSCOPY FOR PANCREATIC ADENOCARCINOMA AND OTHER PERIAMPULLARY TUMORS
Introduction

Most patients with pancreatic ductal adenocarcinoma (PDAC) present with metastatic disease. Ten percent to 15% of patients with radiographically resectable tumors and 30% of patients with locally advanced disease have unresectable disease discovered at laparotomy,[11] most commonly due to radiographically occult liver metastases.[50] SL has become more selective as preoperative imaging has improved and SL yield has decreased.

Benefits of Staging Laparoscopy in Pancreas and Peripancreatic Tumors

Patients with unresectable periampullary tumors discovered during SL spend less time in the hospital postoperatively[2,18] and receive systemic therapy more frequently and sooner than patients with unresectable disease discovered during laparotomy.[1] With improvements in nonoperative therapy for biliary and gastric outlet obstruction, there is a diminishing role for operative biliary and gastric bypass in patients with unresectable periampullary tumors.[51] A study from the Netherlands reported that median survival is equivalent between patients with unresectable periampullary tumors who undergo laparotomy and biliary and/or gastric bypass or SL only; however, patients who only have SL spend less of their remaining survival lifetime admitted to the hospital.[2] A study from MSKCC showed that only 1.9% of patients found to have unresectable disease during SL will require a subsequent laparotomy for palliative biliary or gastric bypass procedures with a median follow-up of 5.9 months, emphasizing the importance of avoiding a nontherapeutic laparotomy.[51,52] A French study of 100 patients with locally unresectable or metastatic PDAC who developed biliary or gastric outlet obstruction reported that nonoperative interventions were greater than 90% successful in relieving jaundice and gastric outlet obstruction, respectively, with only 1 patient requiring a surgical bypass.[51] Taken together, with improvements in nonoperative interventions to relieve biliary and gastric outlet obstruction and equivalent survival in operative and nonoperative bypass procedures, few patients with unresectable PDAC and periampullary tumors will require a laparotomy, emphasizing the importance of avoiding a nontherapeutic laparotomy.

Staging Laparoscopy and Preoperative Imaging

Cross-sectional imaging is used to detect distant metastases and to determine local resectability by assessing the relationship of the tumor with major vascular structures.[5,53,54] A Cochrane Database Systematic Review meta-analysis of 16 studies, including 1146 patients with pancreas and periampullary cancers found to have pathologically confirmed liver or peritoneal metastases, concluded that SL decreases the rate of nontherapeutic laparotomy by 21% compared with CT imaging alone.[17] The meta-analysis found that radiographically resectable tumors as determined by CT were actually unresectable in 41% of cases, and the addition of SL improved the unresectability rate to 20%.

With improvements in imaging technology, detection of smaller metastases and more accurate evaluation of local resectability has limited SL yield; however, radiographically occult metastatic disease is still discovered in some patients during laparotomy.[11,55–59] Early reports of SL in PDAC identified radiographically occult metastases or local unresectability in 31% to 45% of patients.[10,18,60] Contemporary studies determined that SL findings avoided nontherapeutic laparotomy in only 15% of PDAC patients.[11,61,62] Emphasizing the impact of improved imaging on SL, 1045 patients with radiographically resectable pancreas and peripancreatic tumors underwent SL from 1995 to 2005 at MSKCC, and SL yield decreased from 19% to 3% with modern imaging.[11] Owing to the decreasing SL yield, a more selective application of SL has been recommended.[63,64]

Selection of Patients with Pancreas and Periampullary Tumors for Staging Laparoscopy

Modern imaging identifies more patients with locally advanced tumors or subtle findings of metastatic disease,[65] and compared with older studies[10,18,60] that included patients with borderline resectable or locally unresectable tumors who are more likely to harbor radiographically occult metastases, more contemporary studies, including only patients with clearly resectable tumors, report a decreasing SL yield.[11] Identifying those patients with radiographically resectable tumors for whom SL remains valuable is imperative in the current health care climate, whereby responsible resource utilization is paramount.

Tumor histology, location, and size are important determinants of discovering unresectable disease. In the previously discussed study of 1045 patients with radiographically resectable pancreas and periampullary tumors who underwent SL at MSKCC, primary tumor site was the strongest predictor of identifying unresectable disease.[11] SL yield was 14% for PDAC compared with 4% for nonpancreas periampullary tumors. Other studies have reported similar findings.[66–68] In a study from MSKCC, only 10% of patients with nonpancreatic periampullary tumors were found to be unresectable during SL, with the lowest yield for patients with ampullary and duodenal tumors.[69] Tumor location within the pancreas is an important predictor of SL yield, with SL yield higher in body/tail tumors compared with pancreatic head tumors.[11,67,70–72] Tumor size also predicts SL yield.[73,74] In a UK study, 22 of 137 patients had unresectable disease discovered during SL, and only tumor size was found to be predictive, with a 31.3% SL yield when radiographic tumor diameter was greater than 40 mm.[73]

The tumor biomarker CA 19-9, which is typically elevated in patients with metastatic disease,[72] may be used to select patients for SL.[62,71,75,76] In a study from MSKCC, 51 of 262 PDAC patients with available CA 19-9 levels had unresectable disease discovered during SL.[62] The median CA 19-9 level was lower in patients with resectable tumors. A CA 19-9 cutoff value of 130 U/mL was determined to predict discovery of unresectable disease, with unresectable disease detected in 26.4% of patients with CA 19-9 greater than 130 U/mL, compared with 11% of patients with lower levels.

A study from the Massachusetts General Hospital, including 1001 patients with PDAC who underwent SL between 2009 and 2014, found that borderline resectable and locally advanced tumors, CA 19-9 greater than 394 U/L, pancreas body/tail tumors, and no prior neoadjuvant chemotherapy were predictive of discovering metastatic disease during SL.[77] A recent meta-analysis of 24 studies analyzing SL in resectable pancreas cancer found that CA 19-9 ≥150 U/mL and tumor size greater than 3 cm were the most reliable predictors of discovering unresectable disease during SL.[78] A 2008 Consensus Statement recommends selective SL for patients with resectable pancreas cancer: tumors greater than 3 cm located in the pancreatic head, tumors located in the pancreas body/tail, CA 19-9 level greater than 100 U/mL, or equivocal CT findings, and in patients with locally advanced pancreas cancer to rule out occult metastatic disease.[5]

Adjunctive Procedures During Staging Laparoscopy for Pancreas and Periampullary Tumors

Extended laparoscopic dissection, including opening the lesser sac, examining the porta hepatis and the posterior aspect of the liver, and sampling suspicious portal, perigastric, and celiac lymph nodes, may detect additional metastatic disease compared with standard laparoscopy; however, it requires advanced laparoscopic skills.[18,79] Laparoscopic US may also increase the detection of deep liver metastases, assess regional lymphadenopathy,[61,70,80,81] and determine the relationship of the tumor to surrounding vascular structures to inform resectability.[61,70,81,82]

Although rare to be discovered in the absence of macroscopic peritoneal metastasis, SL may also be used to identify microscopic metastatic disease using peritoneal cytology, which is classified as stage IV disease.[37,83] Patients with resected tumors and positive peritoneal cytology have worse median survival than patients with negative cytology[83–87]; however, peritoneal cytology has not gained widespread adoption, and its use in staging PDAC remains undefined. Most pancreas surgeons found no role for peritoneal cytology in the management of pancreas cancer in a recent expert consensus statement.[88]

Summary: Staging Laparoscopy for Pancreatic and Periampullary Tumors

Selective SL is recommended for all radiographically resectable PDAC pancreatic body/tail tumors, pancreatic head tumors greater than 3 cm, CA 19-9 level greater than 100 U/mL, and patients with equivocal or suspicious findings on preoperative cross-sectional imaging,[5] avoiding nontherapeutic laparotomy in up to 25% of patients. SL yield is low for periampullary tumors, and routine SL is not recommended for this patient population.

STAGING LAPAROSCOPY FOR PRIMARY AND SECONDARY LIVER TUMORS
Staging Laparoscopy for Hepatocellular Carcinoma

SL has a limited role in the management of hepatocellular carcinoma (HCC). Early studies reported an SL yield of 16% to 36% and improved resection rates with the use of SL.[89–93] The addition of laparoscopic US improved the resection rate in several studies by identifying inadequate future liver remnant, bilobar metastatic disease, and peritoneal metastasis; however, US failed to identify portal vein and inferior vena cava (IVC) tumor thrombi and local invasion of adjacent organs.[90] A study from MSKCC of 60 patients with potentially operable HCC who underwent SL between 1997 and 2002 determined that liver cirrhosis and radiographic evidence of major vascular invasion or bilobar tumors predicted the likelihood of finding inoperable disease at SL.[92] SL yield was 5% in patients without these factors, 22% with one factor, and 80% in patients with both factors. A study from Hong Kong reported that severe cirrhosis and inadequate future liver remnant were the most common factors precluding resection in 122 patients with potentially operable HCC who underwent SL and laparoscopic US from 2001 to 2007.[93]

Improvements in imaging and patient selection may limit the utility of SL. In a study from the Netherlands, SL yield was 7% in 54 patients with radiographically resectable HCC who underwent preoperative CT using modern scanners and imaging techniques and nuclear medicine scans to measure future liver remnant volumetry and function.[94] Patients with imaging findings of extrahepatic or nodal metastasis, tumor thrombus or invasion of the main portal vein or IVC, and multicentric bilobar disease were excluded. The investigators concluded that modern imaging obviates SL. Indeed, as the accuracy of detecting locally unresectable and multicentric tumors using modern cross-sectional imaging continues to improve[95] and noninvasive means of determining liver fibrosis and cirrhosis proliferate,[96] the role of SL in the management of HCC appears limited.

Staging Laparoscopy for Colorectal Liver Metastasis

Up to 50% of patients with colorectal cancer develop colorectal liver metastasis (CRLM). Resection is appropriate for all medically fit patients without extrahepatic disease when all CRLM can be resected with maintenance of adequate functional liver remnant. Five-year overall survival up to 60% is possible after resection, although many patients present with unresectable disease.[97] SL may identify extrahepatic disease and extensive, multifocal disease precluding resection.

SL yield is low in unselected CRLM patients[89]; however, patients selected to undergo SL based on high-risk features improves SL yield. Jarnagin and colleagues determined that clinical risk score (CRS)[98] correlated with unresectability rates in CRLM patients undergoing SL.[6] Disease-free interval from time of primary tumor discovery to CRLM discovery less than 12 months, greater than 1 CRLM, CRLM size greater than 5 cm, lymph node–positive primary tumor, and carcinoembryonic antigen (CEA) greater than 200 ng/mL were each assigned 1 point, and CRS was calculated by the sum of these factors. Twelve percent of patients with CRS ≤2 had unresectable disease compared with 42% of patients with CRS greater than 2. The association of CRS and unresectability was confirmed in a follow-up study.[99] SL findings did not affect the nontherapeutic laparotomy rate in patients with CRS 0 to 1; however, 11% of CRS 2 to 3 and 24% of CRS 4 to 5 patients avoided a nontherapeutic laparotomy. A study from the United Kingdom including 200 patients with radiographically resectable CRLM reached similar conclusions, with 75% of CRS 4 to 5 patients found to have incurable disease despite extensive preoperative imaging and SL changing the management in 70% of these patients.[100] In another UK study, 77 patients were selected for SL based on high-risk primary tumor factors (T4 tumors, positive circumferential margin, perforation, large bowel obstruction) or multiple, bilobar metastasis, and SL identified unresectable disease in 21%, compared with an unresectability rate of 8% in 338 patients without these factors who proceeded directly to laparotomy.[101] In an Australian study, patients with shorter disease-free intervals, greater number of metastases, and higher CEA levels were selected for SL, and 33% were found to be unresectable.[102] Taken together, SL may detect unresectable disease in some selected patients with high risk CRLM.

Summary: Staging Laparoscopy for Primary and Secondary Liver Tumors

The role of SL in the management of HCC is limited. Selective SL is recommended prior to planned resection in patients with HCC with cirrhosis or radiographic evidence of major vascular invasion or bilobar tumors.

STAGING LAPAROSCOPY FOR BILIARY TRACT TUMORS
Introduction to Staging Laparoscopy for Biliary Tract Tumors

Biliary tract tumors include gallbladder cancer (GBC), intrahepatic cholangiocarcinoma (IHC), hilar cholangiocarcinoma (HC), and distal cholangiocarcinoma. SL for distal cholangiocarcinoma was discussed in the section covering pancreas and periampullary tumors. Most biliary tract tumors are unresectable due to metastasis or local invasion of hilar structures. Despite improvements in preoperative imaging, a significant number of patients with radiographically resectable biliary tract tumors are found to have unresectable disease during attempted curative resection. In a study from MSKCC, unresectable disease was discovered in 153 of 410 patients with potentially resectable hepatobiliary tumors, with SL identifying findings precluding resection in 55%.[89] Patients with unresectable disease who were spared a nontherapeutic laparotomy had a shorter LOS and less morbidity.

Staging Laparoscopy for Gallbladder Cancer

GBC is the most common biliary tract tumor, with a 5-year survival rate of 5%.[103] Most GBC patients present with liver or nodal involvement[104] and unresectable tumors.[105] Despite extensive preoperative imaging, unresectable disease is discovered in a significant number of patients with radiographically resectable GBC during SL or laparotomy.[12,89]

SL prevents nontherapeutic laparotomy in 38% to 62% of GBC patients.[106] In the largest study of SL in GBC, SL identified unresectable disease in 23.2% of 409 patients with radiographically resectable GBC.[12] At laparotomy, an additional 75 (23.8%) patients were found to have unresectable disease, most commonly lymph node involvement (n = 47). SL yield was higher in locally advanced tumors (T3/T4) compared with early tumors (T1/T2), 25.2% versus 10.7% (P = .02). An Italian study including 21 GBC patients reported improved SL yield and accuracy improved from 38.1% to 52.4% and 61.5% to 84.6%, respectively, with laparoscopic US.[107] In a study of 136 GBC patients who had a prior cholecystectomy and presented to MSKCC for definitive resection, 46 patients underwent SL before a planned laparotomy, and SL identified only 2 patients with unresectable disease.[108] In total, 10 patients were found to have disseminated disease, and higher T stage, positive surgical margin, and poor tumor differentiation were found to be independent predictors of disseminated disease.

Overall, routine SL is recommended for GBC patients with an intact gallbladder, and laparoscopic US may improve the detection of unresectable disease. SL may be considered for patients with incidental GBC with T2 or greater tumor, positive surgical margin, or poor tumor differentiation before planned definitive resection.

Staging Laparoscopy for Hilar Cholangiocarcinoma

Surgical management of HC includes resection of the involved intrahepatic and extrahepatic bile ducts and the associated liver parenchyma and caudate lobe.[109] Resectability is determined by lack of extrahepatic disease, adequate functional liver remnant, and ability to reconstruct the biliary tree. Despite improved accuracy of predicting resectability with modern imaging, unresectable disease is discovered in up to 50% of patients at exploration. Local invasion is an important determinant of resectability: tumor extension into bilateral hepatic ducts, unilateral liver atrophy, or biliary extension with contralateral biliary or vascular inflow involvement preclude resection. Selective SL may improve the detection of extrahepatic disease.

In a study from MSKCC, SL yield was 20% to 25% in 59 HC patients with extensive laparoscopic examination.[89] A similar SL yield was reported in a follow-up study, including 56 HC patients who underwent the same extensive laparoscopic exploration.[8] SL accuracy was 80% for detection of peritoneal metastasis, 66% for liver metastasis, and 40% for nodal metastasis. SL failed to identify all locally unresectable tumors. SL yield increased with T stage (T1 9% vs T2/T3 36%) using the Blumgart staging system.[110] Similar findings were reported in a UK study of 82 patients with radiographically resectable HC who underwent SL and laparoscopic US.[14] The yield and accuracy were 41.5% and 53.1%, respectively. Only 20 of 82 (23.8%) underwent resection, and resection rate was correlated with T stage, with 8 of 17 T1 tumors and 1 of 17 T3 tumors resected.

Improved imaging may be decreasing SL yield by improving patient selection. A study from the Netherlands reported an SL yield of 41% and accuracy of 60% in 110 patients.[111] A follow-up study from the same institution reported an SL yield of 14% and accuracy of 32% in 175 patients.[112] An Italian study reported the same 14% SL yield in 35 patients who underwent extensive preoperative imaging.[107] Conversely, a French study reported a 25% SL yield in 20 patients, despite all patients undergoing US and CT and 90% undergoing MRCP.[13] Similarly, a UK study of 100 patients who underwent extensive laparoscopic exploration and US between 1998 and 2011 showed that, despite comprehensive preoperative imaging, SL yield remained at approximately 45% over the course of the study despite improvements in imaging technology.[113]

A study from the Netherlands derived a risk score to improve selection for SL based on preoperative imaging findings.[3] Tumor size $\geq$4.5 cm, bilateral portal vein or main portal vein tumor involvement, and suspected lymph node or extrahepatic metastases were identified as risk factors that predicted positive findings on SL, which was identified in 15% of 273 patients between 2000 and 2015. Patients were grouped into low-, intermediate-, and high-risk groups based on risk score. The unresectability rate in the low- or intermediate-risk groups was less than 30% and ranged from 47.6% to 100% in the high-risk group.

Local invasion of hilar structures is a main determinant of resectability in HC, which is not usually identified during SL. With the ability of improved preoperative imaging to better identify patients with locally advanced tumors, SL should be used selectively in this population.

Staging Laparoscopy for Intrahepatic Cholangiocarcinoma

Few studies are available to guide SL use in the management of IHC. Patients often present with unresectable disease, and resection should be avoided in patients with extrahepatic disease, including nodal involvement beyond regional lymph nodes, bilateral multifocal or multicentric disease, and inadequate future liver remnant.[9] In a California Cancer Registry study including 275 IHC patients, nearly half had multifocal disease, which was associated with worse prognosis compared to patients with isolated tumors.[114] SL identifies unresectable disease in 25% to 36% of patients with radiographically resectable IHC.[13,89]

Expert consensus opinion recommends selective SL in high-risk patients with elevated CA 19-9 levels or preoperative imaging demonstrating multicentric hepatic lesions, questionable vascular invasion, or extrahepatic metastasis.[9]

Summary: Staging Laparoscopy for Biliary Tract Tumors

SL may avoid nontherapeutic laparotomy in some patients with biliary tract tumors. In a meta-analysis of 8 SL studies published since 2000, SL identified unresectable disease in 153 of 472 HC patients and 163 of 590 GBC patients, for a yield of 32.4% and 27.6%, respectively.[115]

Peritoneal and hepatic metastases are more easily detected during SL than nodal involvement or local invasion, which is a main determinant of resectability in biliary tract tumors. GBC patients with an intact gallbladder and those patients with incidentally discovered GBC with $\geq$T2 tumors, positive surgical margins, or poor tumor differentiation should be considered for SL before definitive resection. SL should be considered for HC patients with advanced T stage, larger size, suspected portal venous involvement, or suspected nodal or extrahepatic metastasis. Last, IHC

Table 1
Staging laparoscopy summary

Disease Site	Consideration for SL	References
GEJ and GC	Distal GEJ, ≥T3 GC with peritoneal cytology	30,32,43–46
PDAC	Pancreas body/tail tumors, pancreas head tumors ≥3 cm, CA 19-9 level >100 U/mL	5,11,67,70–74,78
CRLM	High-CRS or high-risk primary tumor	6,99–102
GBC	All patients with intact gallbladder, incidental GBC if ≥T2, positive surgical margin, or poorly differentiated tumor	12,106–108
HC	Tumor ≥4.5 cm, portal vein tumor involvement, suspected lymph node or extrahepatic disease	3
IHC	Elevated CA 19-9, multicentric hepatic lesions, vascular invasion, extrahepatic disease	9

patients with elevated CA 19-9 levels or preoperative imaging demonstrating multicentric hepatic lesions, questionable vascular invasion, or extrahepatic metastasis may benefit from SL.[9]

SUMMARY

SL may avoid a nontherapeutic laparotomy in selected patients with gastric, GEJ, and HPB malignancies. Patients with unresectable disease discovered at SL have a shorter LOS and fewer complications and initiate alternative therapies sooner compared with patients who undergo a nontherapeutic laparotomy. With advances in imaging technology, careful patient selection for SL is imperative (**Table 1**).

REFERENCES

1. Velanovich V, Wollner I, Ajlouni M. Staging laparoscopy promotes increased utilization of postoperative therapy for unresectable intra-abdominal malignancies. J Gastrointest Surg 2000;4(5):542–6.

2. Beenen E, van Roest MH, Sieders E, et al. Staging laparoscopy in patients scheduled for pancreaticoduodenectomy minimizes hospitalization in the remaining life time when metastatic carcinoma is found. Eur J Surg Oncol 2014; 40(8):989–94.

3. Coelen RJ, Ruys AT, Wiggers JK, et al. Development of a risk score to predict detection of metastasized or locally advanced perihilar cholangiocarcinoma at staging laparoscopy. Ann Surg Oncol 2016;23(Suppl 5):904–10.

4. Hashimoto D, Chikamoto A, Sakata K, et al. Staging laparoscopy leads to rapid induction of chemotherapy for unresectable pancreatobiliary cancers. Asian J Endosc Surg 2015;8(1):59–62.

5. Callery MP, Chang KJ, Fishman EK, et al. Pretreatment assessment of resectable and borderline resectable pancreatic cancer: expert consensus statement. Ann Surg Oncol 2009;16(7):1727–33.

6. Jarnagin WR, Conlon K, Bodniewicz J, et al. A clinical scoring system predicts the yield of diagnostic laparoscopy in patients with potentially resectable hepatic colorectal metastases. Cancer 2001;91(6):1121–8.

7. Sarela AI, Lefkowitz R, Brennan MF, et al. Selection of patients with gastric adenocarcinoma for laparoscopic staging. Am J Surg 2006;191(1):134–8.

8. Weber SM, DeMatteo RP, Fong Y, et al. Staging laparoscopy in patients with extrahepatic biliary carcinoma. Analysis of 100 patients. Ann Surg 2002; 235(3):392–9.

9. Weber SM, Ribero D, O'Reilly EM, et al. Intrahepatic cholangiocarcinoma: expert consensus statement. HPB (Oxford) 2015;17(8):669–80.

10. Schachter PP, Avni Y, Gvirz G, et al. The impact of laparoscopy and laparoscopic ultrasound on the management of pancreatic cystic lesions. Arch Surg 2000;135(3):260–4 [discussion: 264].

11. White R, Winston C, Gonen M, et al. Current utility of staging laparoscopy for pancreatic and peripancreatic neoplasms. J Am Coll Surg 2008;206(3):445–50.

12. Agarwal AK, Kalayarasan R, Javed A, et al. The role of staging laparoscopy in primary gall bladder cancer–an analysis of 409 patients: a prospective study to evaluate the role of staging laparoscopy in the management of gallbladder cancer. Ann Surg 2013;258(2):318–23.

13. Goere D, Wagholikar GD, Pessaux P, et al. Utility of staging laparoscopy in subsets of biliary cancers: laparoscopy is a powerful diagnostic tool in patients with intrahepatic and gallbladder carcinoma. Surg Endosc 2006;20(5):721–5.

14. Connor S, Barron E, Wigmore SJ, et al. The utility of laparoscopic assessment in the preoperative staging of suspected hilar cholangiocarcinoma. J Gastrointest Surg 2005;9(4):476–80.

15. Munasinghe A, Kazi W, Taniere P, et al. The incremental benefit of two quadrant lavage for peritoneal cytology at staging laparoscopy for oesophagogastric adenocarcinoma. Surg Endosc 2013;27(11):4049–53.

16. Lee SD, Ryu KW, Eom BW, et al. Prognostic significance of peritoneal washing cytology in patients with gastric cancer. Br J Surg 2012;99(3):397–403.

17. Allen VB, Gurusamy KS, Takwoingi Y, et al. Diagnostic accuracy of laparoscopy following computed tomography (CT) scanning for assessing the resectability with curative intent in pancreatic and periampullary cancer. Cochrane Database Syst Rev 2016;(7):CD009323.

18. Conlon KC, Dougherty E, Klimstra DS, et al. The value of minimal access surgery in the staging of patients with potentially resectable peripancreatic malignancy. Ann Surg 1996;223(2):134–40.

19. Convie L, Thompson RJ, Kennedy R, et al. The current role of staging laparoscopy in oesophagogastric cancer. Ann R Coll Surg Engl 2015;97(2):146–50.

20. Curet MJ. Port site metastases. Am J Surg 2004;187(6):705–12.

21. Shoup M, Brennan MF, Karpeh MS, et al. Port site metastasis after diagnostic laparoscopy for upper gastrointestinal tract malignancies: an uncommon entity. Ann Surg Oncol 2002;9(7):632–6.

22. Velanovich V. The effects of staging laparoscopy on trocar site and peritoneal recurrence of pancreatic cancer. Surg Endosc 2004;18(2):310–3.

23. Ziprin P, Ridgway PF, Peck DH, et al. The theories and realities of port-site metastases: a critical appraisal. J Am Coll Surg 2002;195(3):395–408.

24. Blackshaw GR, Barry JD, Edwards P, et al. Laparoscopy significantly improves the perceived preoperative stage of gastric cancer. Gastric Cancer 2003;6(4): 225–9.

25. Chang L, Stefanidis D, Richardson WS, et al. The role of staging laparoscopy for intraabdominal cancers: an evidence-based review. Surg Endosc 2009;23(2): 231–41.

26. de Graaf GW, Ayantunde AA, Parsons SL, et al. The role of staging laparoscopy in oesophagogastric cancers. Eur J Surg Oncol 2007;33(8):988–92.
27. Kapiev A, Rabin I, Lavy R, et al. The role of diagnostic laparoscopy in the management of patients with gastric cancer. Isr Med Assoc J 2010;12(12):726–8.
28. Muntean V, Mihailov A, Iancu C, et al. Staging laparoscopy in gastric cancer. Accuracy and impact on therapy. J Gastrointestin Liver Dis 2009;18(2):189–95.
29. Yano M, Tsujinaka T, Shiozaki H, et al. Appraisal of treatment strategy by staging laparoscopy for locally advanced gastric cancer. World J Surg 2000;24(9):1130–5 [discussion: 1135–6].
30. Burke EC, Karpeh MS Jr, Conlon KC, et al. Peritoneal lavage cytology in gastric cancer: an independent predictor of outcome. Ann Surg Oncol 1998;5(5):411–5.
31. Power DG, Schattner MA, Gerdes H, et al. Endoscopic ultrasound can improve the selection for laparoscopy in patients with localized gastric cancer. J Am Coll Surg 2009;208(2):173–8.
32. Feussner H, Omote K, Fink U, et al. Pretherapeutic laparoscopic staging in advanced gastric carcinoma. Endoscopy 1999;31(5):342–7.
33. Leake PA, Cardoso R, Seevaratnam R, et al. A systematic review of the accuracy and indications for diagnostic laparoscopy before curative-intent resection of gastric cancer. Gastric Cancer 2012;15(Suppl 1):S38–47.
34. Karanicolas PJ, Elkin EB, Jacks LM, et al. Staging laparoscopy in the management of gastric cancer: a population-based analysis. J Am Coll Surg 2011;213(5):644–51, 651.e1.
35. Bryan RT, Cruickshank NR, Needham SJ, et al. Laparoscopic peritoneal lavage in staging gastric and oesophageal cancer. Eur J Surg Oncol 2001;27(3):291–7.
36. Nath J, Moorthy K, Taniere P, et al. Peritoneal lavage cytology in patients with oesophagogastric adenocarcinoma. Br J Surg 2008;95(6):721–6.
37. Edge SB, Compton CC. The American Joint Committee on Cancer: the 7th edition of the AJCC cancer staging manual and the future of TNM. Ann Surg Oncol 2010;17(6):1471–4.
38. Nekarda H, Gess C, Stark M, et al. Immunocytochemically detected free peritoneal tumour cells (FPTC) are a strong prognostic factor in gastric carcinoma. Br J Cancer 1999;79(3–4):611–9.
39. Katsuragi K, Yashiro M, Sawada T, et al. Prognostic impact of PCR-based identification of isolated tumour cells in the peritoneal lavage fluid of gastric cancer patients who underwent a curative R0 resection. Br J Cancer 2007;97(4):550–6.
40. Kodera Y, Nakanishi H, Yamamura Y, et al. Prognostic value and clinical implications of disseminated cancer cells in the peritoneal cavity detected by reverse transcriptase-polymerase chain reaction and cytology. Int J Cancer 1998;79(4):429–33.
41. Kodera Y, Nakanishi H, Ito S, et al. Quantitative detection of disseminated cancer cells in the greater omentum of gastric carcinoma patients with real-time RT-PCR: a comparison with peritoneal lavage cytology. Gastric Cancer 2002;5(2):69–76.
42. Amin MB, Edge SB, American Joint Committee on Cancer. AJCC cancer staging manual. 8th edition.
43. Bando E, Yonemura Y, Takeshita Y, et al. Intraoperative lavage for cytological examination in 1,297 patients with gastric carcinoma. Am J Surg 1999;178(3):256–62.
44. Ribeiro U Jr, Safatle-Ribeiro AV, Zilberstein B, et al. Does the intraoperative peritoneal lavage cytology add prognostic information in patients with

potentially curative gastric resection? J Gastrointest Surg 2006;10(2):170–6 [discussion: 176–7].

45. Bentrem D, Wilton A, Mazumdar M, et al. The value of peritoneal cytology as a preoperative predictor in patients with gastric carcinoma undergoing a curative resection. Ann Surg Oncol 2005;12(5):347–53.

46. Fukagawa T, Katai H, Saka M, et al. Significance of lavage cytology in advanced gastric cancer patients. World J Surg 2010;34(3):563–8.

47. Cardona K, Zhou Q, Gonen M, et al. Role of repeat staging laparoscopy in locoregionally advanced gastric or gastroesophageal cancer after neoadjuvant therapy. Ann Surg Oncol 2013;20(2):548–54.

48. Mezhir JJ, Shah MA, Jacks LM, et al. Positive peritoneal cytology in patients with gastric cancer: natural history and outcome of 291 patients. Ann Surg Oncol 2010;17(12):3173–80.

49. Lorenzen S, Panzram B, Rosenberg R, et al. Prognostic significance of free peritoneal tumor cells in the peritoneal cavity before and after neoadjuvant chemotherapy in patients with gastric carcinoma undergoing potentially curative resection. Ann Surg Oncol 2010;17(10):2733–9.

50. Valls C, Andia E, Sanchez A, et al. Dual-phase helical CT of pancreatic adenocarcinoma: assessment of resectability before surgery. AJR Am J Roentgenol 2002;178(4):821–6.

51. Maire F, Hammel P, Ponsot P, et al. Long-term outcome of biliary and duodenal stents in palliative treatment of patients with unresectable adenocarcinoma of the head of pancreas. Am J Gastroenterol 2006;101(4):735–42.

52. Espat NJ, Brennan MF, Conlon KC. Patients with laparoscopically staged unresectable pancreatic adenocarcinoma do not require subsequent surgical biliary or gastric bypass. J Am Coll Surg 1999;188(6):649–55 [discussion: 655–7].

53. Reinhold C. Magnetic resonance imaging of the pancreas in 2001. J Gastrointest Surg 2002;6(2):133–5.

54. Kauhanen SP, Komar G, Seppanen MP, et al. A prospective diagnostic accuracy study of 18F-fluorodeoxyglucose positron emission tomography/computed tomography, multidetector row computed tomography, and magnetic resonance imaging in primary diagnosis and staging of pancreatic cancer. Ann Surg 2009;250(6):957–63.

55. Vargas R, Nino-Murcia M, Trueblood W, et al. MDCT in Pancreatic adenocarcinoma: prediction of vascular invasion and resectability using a multiphasic technique with curved planar reformations. AJR Am J Roentgenol 2004;182(2):419–25.

56. Bipat S, Phoa SS, van Delden OM, et al. Ultrasonography, computed tomography and magnetic resonance imaging for diagnosis and determining resectability of pancreatic adenocarcinoma: a meta-analysis. J Comput Assist Tomogr 2005;29(4):438–45.

57. Tapper E, Kalb B, Martin DR, et al. Staging laparoscopy for proximal pancreatic cancer in a magnetic resonance imaging-driven practice: what's it worth? HPB (Oxford) 2011;13(10):732–7.

58. Ellsmere J, Mortele K, Sahani D, et al. Does multidetector-row CT eliminate the role of diagnostic laparoscopy in assessing the resectability of pancreatic head adenocarcinoma? Surg Endosc 2005;19(3):369–73.

59. Shah D, Fisher WE, Hodges SE, et al. Preoperative prediction of complete resection in pancreatic cancer. J Surg Res 2008;147(2):216–20.

60. Jimenez RE, Warshaw AL, Rattner DW, et al. Impact of laparoscopic staging in the treatment of pancreatic cancer. Arch Surg 2000;135(4):409–14 [discussion: 414–5].
61. Doran HE, Bosonnet L, Connor S, et al. Laparoscopy and laparoscopic ultrasound in the evaluation of pancreatic and periampullary tumours. Dig Surg 2004;21(4):305–13.
62. Maithel SK, Maloney S, Winston C, et al. Preoperative CA 19-9 and the yield of staging laparoscopy in patients with radiographically resectable pancreatic adenocarcinoma. Ann Surg Oncol 2008;15(12):3512–20.
63. Pisters PW, Lee JE, Vauthey JN, et al. Laparoscopy in the staging of pancreatic cancer. Br J Surg 2001;88(3):325–37.
64. Mayo SC, Austin DF, Sheppard BC, et al. Evolving preoperative evaluation of patients with pancreatic cancer: does laparoscopy have a role in the current era? J Am Coll Surg 2009;208(1):87–95.
65. Phoa SS, Reeders JW, Rauws EA, et al. Spiral computed tomography for preoperative staging of potentially resectable carcinoma of the pancreatic head. Br J Surg 1999;86(6):789–94.
66. Tilleman EH, Kuiken BW, Phoa SS, et al. Limitation of diagnostic laparoscopy for patients with a periampullary carcinoma. Eur J Surg Oncol 2004;30(6):658–62.
67. Barreiro CJ, Lillemoe KD, Koniaris LG, et al. Diagnostic laparoscopy for periampullary and pancreatic cancer: what is the true benefit? J Gastrointest Surg 2002;6(1):75–81.
68. Vollmer CM, Drebin JA, Middleton WD, et al. Utility of staging laparoscopy in subsets of peripancreatic and biliary malignancies. Ann Surg 2002;235(1):1–7.
69. Brooks AD, Mallis MJ, Brennan MF, et al. The value of laparoscopy in the management of ampullary, duodenal, and distal bile duct tumors. J Gastrointest Surg 2002;6(2):139–45 [discussion: 145–6].
70. Contreras CM, Stanelle EJ, Mansour J, et al. Staging laparoscopy enhances the detection of occult metastases in patients with pancreatic adenocarcinoma. J Surg Oncol 2009;100(8):663–9.
71. Karachristos A, Scarmeas N, Hoffman JP. CA 19-9 levels predict results of staging laparoscopy in pancreatic cancer. J Gastrointest Surg 2005;9(9):1286–92.
72. Fujioka S, Misawa T, Okamoto T, et al. Preoperative serum carcinoembryonic antigen and carbohydrate antigen 19-9 levels for the evaluation of curability and resectability in patients with pancreatic adenocarcinoma. J Hepatobiliary Pancreat Surg 2007;14(6):539–44.
73. Garcea G, Cairns V, Berry DP, et al. Improving the diagnostic yield from staging laparoscopy for periampullary malignancies: the value of preoperative inflammatory markers and radiological tumor size. Pancreas 2012;41(2):233–7.
74. Chiang KC, Lee CH, Yeh CN, et al. A novel role of the tumor size in pancreatic cancer as an ancillary factor for predicting resectability. J Cancer Res Ther 2014;10(1):142–6.
75. Alexakis N, Gomatos IP, Sbarounis S, et al. High serum CA 19-9 but not tumor size should select patients for staging laparoscopy in radiological resectable pancreas head and peri-ampullary cancer. Eur J Surg Oncol 2015;41(2):265–9.
76. Connor S, Bosonnet L, Alexakis N, et al. Serum CA19-9 measurement increases the effectiveness of staging laparoscopy in patients with suspected pancreatic malignancy. Dig Surg 2005;22(1–2):80–5.
77. Fong ZV, Alvino DML, Fernandez-Del Castillo C, et al. Reappraisal of Staging Laparoscopy for Patients with Pancreatic Adenocarcinoma: A Contemporary Analysis of 1001 Patients. Ann Surg Oncol 2017;24(11):3203–11.

78. De Rosa A, Cameron IC, Gomez D. Indications for staging laparoscopy in pancreatic cancer. HPB (Oxford) 2016;18(1):13–20.

79. Schnelldorfer T, Gagnon AI, Birkett RT, et al. Staging laparoscopy in pancreatic cancer: a potential role for advanced laparoscopic techniques. J Am Coll Surg 2014;218(6):1201–6.

80. Reddy KR, Levi J, Livingstone A, et al. Experience with staging laparoscopy in pancreatic malignancy. Gastrointest Endosc 1999;49(4 Pt 1):498–503.

81. Callery MP, Strasberg SM, Doherty GM, et al. Staging laparoscopy with laparoscopic ultrasonography: optimizing resectability in hepatobiliary and pancreatic malignancy. J Am Coll Surg 1997;185(1):33–9.

82. Minnard EA, Conlon KC, Hoos A, et al. Laparoscopic ultrasound enhances standard laparoscopy in the staging of pancreatic cancer. Ann Surg 1998;228(2): 182–7.

83. Makary MA, Warshaw AL, Centeno BA, et al. Implications of peritoneal cytology for pancreatic cancer management. Arch Surg 1998;133(4):361–5.

84. Clark CJ, Traverso LW. Positive peritoneal lavage cytology is a predictor of worse survival in locally advanced pancreatic cancer. Am J Surg 2010;199(5): 657–62.

85. Ferrone CR, Haas B, Tang L, et al. The influence of positive peritoneal cytology on survival in patients with pancreatic adenocarcinoma. J Gastrointest Surg 2006;10(10):1347–53.

86. Leach SD, Rose JA, Lowy AM, et al. Significance of peritoneal cytology in patients with potentially resectable adenocarcinoma of the pancreatic head. Surgery 1995;118(3):472–8.

87. Yamada S, Fujii T, Kanda M, et al. Value of peritoneal cytology in potentially resectable pancreatic cancer. Br J Surg 2013;100(13):1791–6.

88. Lutz MP, Zalcberg JR, Ducreux M, et al. 3rd St. Gallen EORTC Gastrointestinal Cancer Conference: Consensus recommendations on controversial issues in the primary treatment of pancreatic cancer. Eur J Cancer 2017;79:41–9.

89. D'Angelica M, Fong Y, Weber S, et al. The role of staging laparoscopy in hepatobiliary malignancy: prospective analysis of 401 cases. Ann Surg Oncol 2003; 10(2):183–9.

90. Lo CM, Lai EC, Liu CL, et al. Laparoscopy and laparoscopic ultrasonography avoid exploratory laparotomy in patients with hepatocellular carcinoma. Ann Surg 1998;227(4):527–32.

91. Lo CM, Fan ST, Liu CL, et al. Determining resectability for hepatocellular carcinoma: the role of laparoscopy and laparoscopic ultrasonography. J Hepatobiliary Pancreat Surg 2000;7(3):260–4.

92. Weitz J, D'Angelica M, Jarnagin W, et al. Selective use of diagnostic laparoscopy before planned hepatectomy for patients with hepatocellular carcinoma. Surgery 2004;135(3):273–81.

93. Lai EC, Tang CN, Ha JP, et al. The evolving influence of laparoscopy and laparoscopic ultrasonography on patients with hepatocellular carcinoma. Am J Surg 2008;196(5):736–40.

94. Hoekstra LT, Bieze M, Busch OR, et al. Staging laparoscopy in patients with hepatocellular carcinoma: is it useful? Surg Endosc 2013;27(3):826–31.

95. Tang A, Bashir MR, Corwin MT, et al. Evidence supporting LI-RADS major features for CT- and MR imaging-based diagnosis of hepatocellular carcinoma: a systematic review. Radiology 2018;286(1):29–48.

96. Barr RG, Ferraioli G, Palmeri ML, et al. Elastography assessment of liver fibrosis: society of radiologists in ultrasound consensus conference statement. Ultrasound Q 2016;32(2):94–107.
97. Misiakos EP, Karidis NP, Kouraklis G. Current treatment for colorectal liver metastases. World J Gastroenterol 2011;17(36):4067–75.
98. Fong Y, Fortner J, Sun RL, et al. Clinical score for predicting recurrence after hepatic resection for metastatic colorectal cancer: analysis of 1001 consecutive cases. Ann Surg 1999;230(3):309–18 [discussion: 318–21].
99. Grobmyer SR, Fong Y, D'Angelica M, et al. Diagnostic laparoscopy before planned hepatic resection for colorectal metastases. Arch Surg 2004;139(12): 1326–30.
100. Mann CD, Neal CP, Metcalfe MS, et al. Clinical Risk Score predicts yield of staging laparoscopy in patients with colorectal liver metastases. Br J Surg 2007; 94(7):855–9.
101. Pilkington SA, Rees M, Peppercorn D, et al. Laparoscopic staging in selected patients with colorectal liver metastases as a prelude to liver resection. HPB (Oxford) 2007;9(1):58–63.
102. Metcalfe MS, Close JS, Iswariah H, et al. The value of laparoscopic staging for patients with colorectal metastases. Arch Surg 2003;138(7):770–2.
103. Hundal R, Shaffer EA. Gallbladder cancer: epidemiology and outcome. Clin Epidemiol 2014;6:99–109.
104. Ito H, Ito K, D'Angelica M, et al. Accurate staging for gallbladder cancer: implications for surgical therapy and pathological assessment. Ann Surg 2011; 254(2):320–5.
105. Sheth S, Bedford A, Chopra S. Primary gallbladder cancer: recognition of risk factors and the role of prophylactic cholecystectomy. Am J Gastroenterol 2000;95(6):1402–10.
106. Aloia TA, Jarufe N, Javle M, et al. Gallbladder cancer: expert consensus statement. HPB (Oxford) 2015;17(8):681–90.
107. Russolillo N, D'Eletto M, Langella S, et al. Role of laparoscopic ultrasound during diagnostic laparoscopy for proximal biliary cancers: a single series of 100 patients. Surg Endosc 2016;30(3):1212–8.
108. Butte JM, Gonen M, Allen PJ, et al. The role of laparoscopic staging in patients with incidental gallbladder cancer. HPB (Oxford) 2011;13(7):463–72.
109. Mansour JC, Aloia TA, Crane CH, et al. Hilar cholangiocarcinoma: expert consensus statement. HPB (Oxford) 2015;17(8):691–9.
110. Jarnagin WR, Fong Y, DeMatteo RP, et al. Staging, resectability, and outcome in 225 patients with hilar cholangiocarcinoma. Ann Surg 2001;234(4):507–17 [discussion: 517–9].
111. Tilleman EH, de Castro SM, Busch OR, et al. Diagnostic laparoscopy and laparoscopic ultrasound for staging of patients with malignant proximal bile duct obstruction. J Gastrointest Surg 2002;6(3):426–30 [discussion: 430–1].
112. Ruys AT, Busch OR, Gouma DJ, et al. Staging laparoscopy for hilar cholangiocarcinoma: is it still worthwhile? Ann Surg Oncol 2011;18(9):2647–53.
113. Barlow AD, Garcea G, Berry DP, et al. Staging laparoscopy for hilar cholangiocarcinoma in 100 patients. Langenbecks Arch Surg 2013;398(7):983–8.
114. Raoof M, Dumitra S, Ituarte PHG, et al. Development and validation of a prognostic score for intrahepatic cholangiocarcinoma. JAMA Surg 2017;152(5): e170117.
115. Tian Y, Liu L, Yeolkar NV, et al. Diagnostic role of staging laparoscopy in a subset of biliary cancers: a meta-analysis. ANZ J Surg 2017;87(1–2):22–7.

Minimally Invasive Surgery for Palliation

Jordan M. Cloyd, MD

KEYWORDS

- Minimally invasive surgery • Robotic • Laparoscopic • Endoscopic • Bypass
- Palliative

KEY POINTS

- Palliative care is the multidisciplinary focus on patient symptoms and quality of life. Although many symptoms can be addressed with pharmacologic or behavioral remedies, palliative surgery is occasionally needed for maximal relief.
- Minimally invasive surgery is an optimal platform for which to perform palliative surgery because of its emphasis on reduced postoperative pain and faster recovery.
- Upper gastrointestinal and hepatopancreatobiliary malignancies commonly lead to gastric outlet obstruction and jaundice, which can be managed endoscopically or surgically in a minimally invasive fashion.
- Lower gastrointestinal malignancies can lead to obstruction, bleeding, and ascites for which minimally invasive strategies are available.
- Minimally invasive surgical palliation may also be indicated in the management of complications of therapy for cancer, in addition to complications of the cancer itself.

INTRODUCTION

Palliative care is the multidisciplinary focus on patient symptoms with the goal of preservation or improvement in quality of life (QOL). Cancer, especially in its late stages, can lead to a multitude of devastating physical and psychosocial symptoms that significantly impede the quality and dignity of patients' lives. Although not mutually exclusive to curative-intent therapies, palliative care is most often prioritized in patients in whom symptoms are worsened because of progressive and/or metastatic disease and not amenable to standard curative-based treatments (eg, resection of the offending tumor). Paradoxically, early palliative care consultation, in addition to improvements in mood and QOL, has been shown to result in longer survival durations.[1] A focus on palliative care begins with a comprehensive understanding of a patient's symptoms, priorities, and goals of care. Although many symptoms can be addressed

Disclosure Statement: The author reports no relevant disclosures.
Department of Surgery, The Ohio State University, 410 West 10th Avenue, N-907, Columbus, OH 43210, USA
E-mail address: Jordan.cloyd@osumc.edu

with pharmacologic or behavioral remedies, not infrequently interventional procedures are required for optimal relief.

Just as oncologic surgery is an opportunity to cure patients of their cancer, palliative surgery is an opportunity to cure patients of their symptoms. However, the decision to perform palliative surgery in a patient with metastatic incurable cancer must be made thoughtfully as part of a multidisciplinary evaluation that carefully weighs the advantages and disadvantages of surgery. In aiming to relieve one's symptoms, surgery invariably leads to other at least transient postoperative symptoms (ie, pain, nausea, fatigue, etc.). In addition, for most operations a period of time off all cytotoxic treatments is required, thereby delaying or impeding the receipt of (potentially) life-extending treatments. Both of these factors become more pronounced in the setting of postoperative complications.

Based on these considerations, minimally invasive surgery (MIS) is perhaps the optimal platform for which to perform palliative surgery. MIS is associated with reduced postoperative pain and faster recovery, both important factors for patients who prioritize symptom control and QOL. Furthermore, oncologic outcomes such as margin status and lymph node yield, 2 factors often mentioned as potential concerns of MIS, are less important in the palliative setting. As the systemic and locoregional treatment options continue to evolve and improve, even for the most aggressive malignancies, the number of patients who require surgical palliation of their diseases will continue to increase. In this article, the authors discuss common symptoms associated with solid organ malignancies as well as the minimally invasive approaches to surgical palliation.

UPPER GASTROINTESTINAL AND HEPATOPANCREATOBILIARY MALIGNANCIES
Gastric Outlet Obstruction

Gastric outlet obstruction (GOO) is a common condition among patients with pancreatic, periampullary, and gastric neoplasms, which can lead to debilitating pain, distension, nausea, vomiting, and oral intolerance. Furthermore, the weight loss and hypoalbuminemia associated with poor oral intake interferes with the receipt of oncologic therapy. Addressing this condition is an important goal of the surgical oncologist. A variety of interventions can be used, the selection of which depends on the goals of the patient, current therapies, previous operations, and patient performance status. For patients with poor performance status and short life expectancy, a decompressing gastrostomy tube can provide adequate relief, avoid the discomfort of a nasogastric tube, and permit discharge from the hospital. Gastrostomy tubes can be placed under interventional, endoscopic, or laparoscopic guidance depending on the particular situation.

For patients with reasonable life expectancy but who are not good surgical candidates (eg, comorbidities, current systemic chemotherapy, etc), endoscopic stent placement has been shown to be a safe and effective means of improving oral intake. Duodenal stents typically measure 60 to 90 mm in length, may be covered or uncovered, and are placed under endoscopic and fluoroscopic guidance. A systematic review of institutional series demonstrated a pooled technical success rate of 97% and clinical success rate of 87%.[2] Mean time to clinical improvement was less than 4 days, no procedure-related mortality was observed, and there was a very low rate of short-term complications. Nevertheless, long-term complications of occlusion or migration occurred in approximately 25% of cases.

Minimally invasive gastrojejunostomy (GJ) should be strongly considered for patients with GOO, good performance status, and unresectable disease. Multiple series have demonstrated MIS GJ to be safe and feasible in patients with unresectable gastrointestinal malignancies even among those with previous abdominal surgery and/or who have failed previous endoscopic stenting.[3–5] Compared with open GJ, laparoscopic GJ led to a decreased time to oral intake and shorter length of hospital stay in one randomized controlled trial.[6] Laparoscopic GJ can be performed in a split-leg, low lithotomy, or supine position. With the patient in the supine position, 3 to 4 laparoscopic trocars are placed under direct vision and the abdomen is explored. With the transverse colon reflected cephalad, a loop of proximal jejunum is identified and approximated to the antrum of the stomach. After making a separate enterotomy and gastrotomy, the GJ is made using a 45- to 60-mm linear endoscopic stapler. The opening is inspected to examine for bleeding and then closed using intracorporeal sutures. Alternatively, a sutured GJ anastomosis can be performed, which may be facilitated using the robotic platform (**Fig. 1**). Whereas some advocate performing an antecolic GJ to reduce the proximity of the anastomosis to tumor, others prefer a retrocolic, isoperistaltic GJ in order to minimize the chances of delayed gastric emptying.

The decision to perform endoscopic stenting versus surgical GJ has been the subject of multiple retrospective comparisons and a few small randomized controlled trials.[7,8] In general, although endoscopic stent is associated with shorter time to oral intake and reduced initial length of hospital stay, surgical GJ is associated with more durable results and reduced need for reintervention.[9] One important note is that most of the studies directly comparing these 2 treatment modalities included open GJs, whereas the inclusion of MIS GJ may have minimized differences between short-term outcomes observed in the endoscopic versus surgical arms.

Jaundice

Obstructive jaundice from upper gastrointestinal and hepatopancreatobiliary malignancies is a disabling condition associated with symptomatic pruritus, malabsorption, coagulopathy, and risk of cholangitis and cholestatic liver dysfunction. Similar to GOO, biliary obstruction can be managed surgically or endoscopically. Although both are effective at relieving jaundice, given the higher morbidity associated with operative interventions, endoscopic biliary stent placement is typically the primary approach for most patients. In early clinical trials, biliary stents were associated with a higher incidence of recurrent jaundice and need for reintervention compared with biliary bypass.[10,11] However, these studies were performed with plastic stents that have a much higher rate of failure and need for exchange. Self-expanding metal stents (SEMS), both covered and uncovered, are associated with fewer complications, do not eliminate the potential for future pancreatoduodenectomy if indicated, and are the most cost-effective solution for biliary obstruction.[12] One large randomized controlled trial demonstrated a median time to recurrent biliary obstruction of

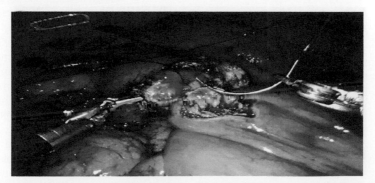

Fig. 1. Example of robotic gastrojejunostomy using two-layer sutured technique.

711 days with the use of uncovered SEMS compared with 357 days for partially covered SEMS, suggesting uncovered metal stents should be primarily used.[13]

In rare situations outside of the prophylactic scenario performed during an aborted pancreatoduodenectomy, surgical biliary bypass may be indicated. Example scenarios where a surgical biliary bypass could be required include the following: the inability to cannulize the biliary tree, the hospital does not have the expertise to perform a "rendez-vouz" procedure, or the patient has a history of roux-en-y gastric bypass preventing endoscopic access to the bile duct. Multiple surgical approaches to biliary obstruction exist without strong evidence favoring one over other. Simply, biliary bypass can occur via either the common bile duct (choledocho- or hepatico-) or the gallbladder (cholecysto-) to either the duodenum or the jejunum, the latter via either a loop or roux-en-y fashion. These operations can be performed via traditional laparoscopy or robotic-assisted laparoscopy.

In terms of minimally invasive approaches, cholecystojejunostomy is the simplest to perform. However, previous reports demonstrated high failure rates due to malignant obstruction of the cystic duct.[14] Nevertheless, those patients with a normal gallbladder and malignancy far from the cystic duct junction could be considered for a cholecystojejunostomy. The procedure is performed in the supine position with 4 laparoscopic trocars in a triangulated position over the location of planned anastomosis. A loop of jejunum approximately 30 cm distal to the ligament of Treitz is selected and brought antecolic to the right upper quadrant. After placing 2 stay sutures, and making a separate enterotomy and cholecystectomy, an anastomosis is fashioned using a 30-mm linear endoscopic stapler. Finally, the common opening is closed with intracorporeal sutures.

Although cholecystojejunostomy is an option, given its overall low morbidity, excellent durability, reduced risk of cholangitis, and relative simplicity to perform, a roux-en-y hepaticojejunostomy should be the preferred surgical approach to biliary obstruction when technically feasible. With the patient in the left lateral position and the coastal margin elevated, 4 laparoscopic trocars are placed. The jejunum is divided approximately 30 cm distal to the ligament of Treitz and the small bowel mesentery elongated such that a roux limb is brought to the right upper quadrant in a retrocolic or antecolic fashion. The common bile duct (CBD) is dissected and then divided. Although frozen section confirms the absence of malignancy at the site of anastomosis, the distal end of the CBD is oversewn. Next, a choledochojejunostomy is formed using absorbable monofilament suture in a running fashion for the posterior layer and interrupted fashion for the anterior layer (**Fig. 2**). Alternatively, the CBD can be opened longitudinally and a

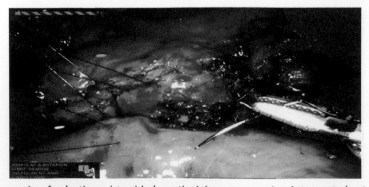

Fig. 2. Example of robotic end-to-side hepaticojejunostomy using interrupted sutures.

side-to-side choledochojejunsotomy created. Finally, a jejunojejunostomy is created in the surgeon's preferred fashion at a location that permits a roux limb of approximately 45 cm.

Pain

Most of the patients with unresectable pancreatic ductal adenocarcinoma or other periampullary cancers experience significant pain for which the mainstay is multimodality analgesics. However, because tumor infiltration of the celiac plexus is a common cause of significant pain, celiac nerve plexus block is a minimally invasive procedure that reduces patient-reported pain and leads to less usage of opioid analgesics.[15] Celiac nerve plexus block can be performed via surgical, percutaneous, or endoscopic ultrasound (EUS)-guided approaches. Few studies have directly compared percutaneous with EUS-guided approaches, those that were performed in patients with chronic pancreatitis and showed no difference in outcomes.[16] Meta-analyses of EUS-guided celiac neurolysis suggest low risk of complications and a high success rate.[17]

A landmark trial by Lillemoe and colleagues[18] studied the efficacy of intraoperative celiac neurolysis using 50% ethanol among patients who were found at the time of laparotomy to be unresectable. Patients randomized to celiac nerve plexus block had significantly improved pain scores at 2, 4, and 6 months after surgery. With the advent of percutaneous and EUS-guided approaches, the need for surgical celiac neurolysis has waned. However, for patients who are not candidates for either of these approaches, laparoscopic celiac plexus block is safe, simple, and effective.[19]

Dysphagia

Dysphagia is the most common presenting sign of esophageal and gastroesophageal junction cancers but often signifies advanced stage disease. Fortunately, multiple endoscopic techniques are available to palliate patients in a minimally invasive fashion. Esophageal dilation has a role in the transient relief of malignant stenosis; however, the results are effective for only several weeks, so other more durable solutions are needed. Similar to their use in the duodenum, SEMS provide symptomatic relief in up to 95% of patients, despite the 20% to 40% rate of complications that include obstruction, migration, and fistulization. Other endoscopic treatments such as laser recanalization using yttrium aluminum garnet (YAG) or photodynamic therapy (PDT) provide transient relief of esophageal stenosis and can be repeated every 4 to 8 weeks. Finally, palliative chemotherapy and chemoradiation therapy can improve symptoms in up to 90% of patients.

The importance of maintaining enteral nutrition should be emphasized. If attempts at resolving esophageal stenosis fail to improve oral intake adequately, other forms of enteral nutrition should be pursued. Laparoscopic jejunostomy feeding tube placement is the preferred method especially in those who may be candidates for resection where preservation of the gastric conduit is important. A variety of methods have been described with no direct studies showing superiority of one method over others. Most descriptions entail percutaneous passage of a feeding tube into the proximal jejunum; placement of a purse-string suture or Witzel tunnel using intracorporeal suturing; and securement to the abdominal wall using either intracorporeal suturing, a transfacial suture passer, or tacks.[20–22] Alternatively, several commercial kits are available that rely on a Seldinger technique with serial dilators to perform needle tube jejunostomy. MIS feeding jejunostomy tube placement is safe, feasible, and associated with a low rate of complications.[21]

LOWER GASTROINTESTINAL CANCER
Obstruction

Patients who present with colonic obstruction represent a surgical emergency. Disadvantages to emergency surgery in this setting, however, include a dilated proximal colon, malnourishment, lack of proper bowel preparation, and the possible concurrent receipt of cytotoxic chemotherapy. For these reasons and others, endoscopic placement of SEMS is an attractive alternative. A systematic review of 1785 patients undergoing colonic stent placement found the median technical and clinical success rates were 96% and 92%, respectively with specific complications (eg, perforation, migration) ranging from 5% to 12%.[23] The disadvantages of colonic stent placement include technical limitations (eg, hepatic or splenic flexure), the inability to receive antiangiogenic agents such as bevacizumab, and their short durability. For this reason, most consider the use of colonic stent only as a bridge to surgery or in patients with limited prognosis.

Laparoscopic resection or colostomy is a viable option for patients who fail or are not good candidates for colonic stent placement. Laparoscopic loop sigmoid colostomy is the preferred procedure for obstructing rectal cancers and is frequently considered before systemic chemotherapy and/or chemoradiation. The operation can be performed with as few as one port in addition to the colostomy site. Minimally invasive transverse colostomy, cecostomy, or ileostomy can also be performed based on the location of obstruction. Surgical bypass via laparoscopic ileocolostomy can also be considered in well-selected patients with right-sided colonic obstruction. Finally, minimally invasive colostomy may be an appropriate palliative option for patients with significant rectal pain, bleeding, or fistulization.

Ascites

Malignant ascites occurs most commonly in the setting of metastatic ovarian or colorectal cancer but is also seen in a variety of other malignancies. Patients with symptomatic malignant ascites experience poor QOL secondary to abdominal pain, distension, nausea, vomiting, and anorexia. Because medical management alone is rarely effective, palliative interventions are indicated. Percutaneous paracentesis is a safe, effective, and reproducible procedure that rapidly evacuates ascites. Because many patients require multiple paracenteses, placement of a tunneled drainage catheter is an effective and convenient method for repeated intermittent drainage of ascites. Previous cost analyses have demonstrated that tunneled catheters are cost-effective once a patient has received approximately 9 paracenteses.[24]

Because malignant ascites develops in the setting of peritoneal carcinomatosis, it has been observed that patients who undergo hyperthermic intraperitoneal chemotherapy (HIPEC) have improvements in their ascites even when incomplete cytoreduction is performed. With the ability to perform HIPEC in a minimally invasive fashion, this is a reasonable option for patients with malignant ascites, disabling symptoms, and good performance status. Laparoscopic HIPEC can be performed with or without cytoreductive surgery. For example, debulking of peritoneal disease (eg, omentectomy) may contribute significantly to the production of malignant ascites. Regardless, 2 large catheters are placed into the upper abdomen under direct visualization and positioned under the left and right hemidiaphragms. The external portions of the catheters are connected to a closed circuit system for intraperitoneal chemotherapy administration. No standardized chemotherapy regimen, dose, duration of perfusion, or intraperitoneal temperature has been established. Despite this heterogeneity, most patients experience resolution of their symptoms with a low incidence of complications.[25–27]

OTHER SCENARIOS
Bleeding Metastases

With recent breakthroughs in immuno-oncology, patients with metastatic melanoma are living significantly longer. The need therefore for palliative interventions in patients with metastatic melanoma will only increase. For example, melanoma is the most common metastasis to the small bowel and frequently presents with gastrointestinal bleeding. This scenario can significantly impair QOL, leading to frequent emergency room visits, hospitalization, and red blood cell transfusions. Therefore, palliative surgery, in appropriate surgical candidates, is clearly indicated.

Except in the patient with multiple prior abdominal operations, small bowel resection can occur in a minimally invasive fashion. The offending metastasis can typically be located on preoperative imaging and should be visible and palpable with laparoscopic instruments. For patients with obvious small bowel melanoma metastases, preoperative colonoscopy and/or endoscopy is not routinely required to rule out other sources of bleeding. In addition, if the offending metastasis can be definitively identified, then resection of concurrent metastases at the time of surgery is not required. Furthermore, wide mesenteric lymph node dissection is not required. There is some evidence to suggest that surgery can be safely performed in the setting of checkpoint inhibitors and probably restarted shortly after surgery.[28] The long-term outcomes of surgery for bleeding metastases are unknown but palliative surgery for metastatic melanoma is well established.[29]

Other gastrointestinal as well as pulmonary, endocrine, gynecologic, and genitourinary malignancies can present with bleeding as well. Many of these tumors can be palliated using minimally invasive approaches such as endoscopy, cystoscopy, or colonoscopy. Control of bleeding with electrocautery, injection of epinephrine, clip application, and other maneuvers is frequently successful. Surgical intervention when these efforts fail should be made on a case-by-case basis weighing the risks of surgery, the health and performance status of the patient, their life expectancy, the acuity and severity of the bleeding, and concurrent oncologic therapies.

Malignant Pleural Effusions

Malignant pleural effusions are a common morbid condition among patients with primary and metastatic lung cancers. Many patients with malignant pleural effusions experience significant dyspnea on exertion, cough, or chest discomfort. Although the median life expectancy of patients with malignant effusions is less than 6 months, palliative interventions are indicated for those with significant symptoms. A large-volume thoracentesis, typically required anyways for confirmation of diagnosis, is used to assess the symptomatic response to treatment. For those who experience resolution or improvement of their symptoms, further minimally invasive interventions are indicated. Note that up to 50% of patients with symptomatic malignant pleural effusions will not improve because of lung deconditioning, comorbid conditions, or incomplete reexpansion of the lung.

For patients whose symptoms respond to thoracentesis but have rapid return of pleural effusions, several management options exist. For reasonably fit patients without entrapped lung, video-assisted thoracoscopic surgery (VATS) pleurodesis is effective at reducing the recurrence of pleural effusions. Talc pleurodesis can also be instilled via an indwelling chest tube; however, there is some evidence that VATS-assisted pleurodesis may be more effective.[30] On the other hand, tunneled pleural catheters are becoming the preferred modality for recurrent malignant pleural effusions by many physicians. Pleural catheters can be safely placed on an outpatient basis with a low risk of procedural complications. They can technically be removed, but given the poor prognosis of this condition, they rarely are.[31]

Complications of Therapy

Palliative surgery should address not only complications of the cancer but also complications from treatment for the cancer. It is well known that cytotoxic therapies have disabling side effects, but they also can lead to life-threatening complications in some patients. Palliative surgery should be considered in the appropriate context for either of these reasons and, when possible, be performed in a minimally invasive fashion. Many such examples exist. Patients who develop bowel perforations on checkpoint inhibitors or targeted therapies may need emergent surgery. Those who develop disabling proctitis or ureteral fibrosis as complications of radiation may benefit from diverting colostomy or ureteral stents, respectively. Patients receiving somatostatin analogues for metastatic neuroendocrine tumors often develop symptomatic cholelithiasis, and palliative cholecystectomy should be considered. As with all scenarios in this article, a multidisciplinary, patient-centered approach should be used to guide any decision-making with regard to performing palliative surgery.

SUMMARY

By definition, palliative surgery shifts the goals of therapy from a curative-intent focus to an emphasis on symptoms and QOL. As oncologic therapies improve and patients with advanced stage cancer are living longer, the importance of effective interventions for palliation will only continue to increase. Indeed, the importance of palliative surgery is increasingly being recognized in formal training programs. For example, Hospice and Palliative Medicine (HPM) has been a recognized medical subspecialty by the American Board of Medical Specialties since 2006 and the American Board of Surgery offers board certification in HPM to surgeons who complete a 1-year ACGME-approved fellowship.[32]

The focus of MIS on reduced pain and faster recovery aligns well with the goals of palliative care. As discussed in this article, minimally invasive approaches can be safely and effectively used to address several common complications of solid organ malignancies. On the other hand, palliative surgery is critical in addressing the complications of therapy as well. Importantly, palliative care must be delivered as part of an interdisciplinary team with representatives from medical oncology, radiation oncology, surgical oncology, HPM, nursing, pharmacy, and others. Furthermore, although many issues can be addressed via pharmacologic, endoscopic, or other nonoperative methods (eg, radiation, chemotherapy, interventional procedures), when palliative surgery is indicated, it can nearly always be performed in a minimally invasive fashion. This patient-centered, minimally invasive approach will not only help alleviate disabling symptoms and improve QOL but also minimize the pain and adverse effects of the surgical intervention itself.

REFERENCES

1. Temel JS, Greer JA, Muzikansky A, et al. Early palliative care for patients with metastatic non-small-cell lung cancer. N Engl J Med 2010;363(8): 733–42.
2. Dormann A, Meisner S, Verin N, et al. Self-expanding metal stents for gastroduodenal malignancies: systematic review of their clinical effectiveness. Endoscopy 2004;36(6):543–50.

3. Kazanjian KK, Reber HA, Hines OJ. Laparoscopic gastrojejunostomy for gastric outlet obstruction in pancreatic cancer. Am Surg 2004;70(10):910–3.
4. Choi Y-B. Laparoscopic gatrojejunostomy for palliation of gastric outlet obstruction in unresectable gastric cancer. Surg Endosc 2002;16(11):1620–6.
5. Zhang LP, Tabrizian P, Nguyen S, et al. Laparoscopic gastrojejunostomy for the treatment of gastric outlet obstruction. JSLS 2011;15(2):169–73.
6. Navarra G, Musolino C, Venneri A, et al. Palliative antecolic isoperistaltic gastro-jejunostomy: a randomized controlled trial comparing open and laparoscopic approaches. Surg Endosc 2006;20(12):1831–4.
7. Mehta S, Hindmarsh A, Cheong E, et al. Prospective randomized trial of laparoscopic gastrojejunostomy versus duodenal stenting for malignant gastric outflow obstruction. Surg Endosc 2006;20(2):239–42.
8. Jeurnink SM, Steyerberg EW, van Hooft JE, et al. Surgical gastrojejunostomy or endoscopic stent placement for the palliation of malignant gastric outlet obstruction (SUSTENT study): a multicenter randomized trial. Gastrointest Endosc 2010; 71(3):490–9.
9. Bian S-B, Shen W-S, Xi H-Q, et al. Palliative therapy for gastric outlet obstruction caused by unresectable gastric cancer: a meta-analysis comparison of gastrojejunostomy with endoscopic stenting. Chin Med J (Engl) 2016;129(9):1113–21.
10. Smith AC, Dowsett JF, Russell RC, et al. Randomised trial of endoscopic stenting versus surgical bypass in malignant low bileduct obstruction. Lancet 1994; 344(8938):1655–60.
11. Speer AG, Cotton PB, Russell RC, et al. Randomised trial of endoscopic versus percutaneous stent insertion in malignant obstructive jaundice. Lancet 1987; 2(8550):57–62.
12. Almadi MA, Barkun A, Martel M. Plastic vs. self-expandable metal stents for palliation in malignant biliary obstruction: a series of meta-analyses. Am J Gastroenterol 2017;112(2):260–73.
13. Telford JJ, Carr-Locke DL, Baron TH, et al. A randomized trial comparing uncovered and partially covered self-expandable metal stents in the palliation of distal malignant biliary obstruction. Gastrointest Endosc 2010;72(5):907–14.
14. Sarfeh IJ, Rypins EB, Jakowatz JG, et al. A prospective, randomized clinical investigation of cholecystoenterostomy and choledochoenterostomy. Am J Surg 1988;155(3):411–4.
15. Arcidiacono PG, Calori G, Carrara S, et al. Celiac plexus block for pancreatic cancer pain in adults. Cochrane Database Syst Rev 2011;3:CD007519.
16. Moura RN, De Moura EGH, Bernardo WM, et al. Endoscopic-ultrasound versus percutaneous-guided celiac plexus block for chronic pancreatitis pain. A systematic review and meta-analysis. Rev Gastroenterol Peru 2015;35(4):333–41.
17. Puli SR, Reddy JBK, Bechtold ML, et al. EUS-guided celiac plexus neurolysis for pain due to chronic pancreatitis or pancreatic cancer pain: a meta-analysis and systematic review. Dig Dis Sci 2009;54(11):2330–7.
18. Lillemoe KD, Cameron JL, Kaufman HS, et al. Chemical splanchnicectomy in patients with unresectable pancreatic cancer. A prospective randomized trial. Ann Surg 1993;217(5):447–55 [discussion: 456–7].
19. Allen PJ, Chou J, Janakos M, et al. Prospective evaluation of laparoscopic celiac plexus block in patients with unresectable pancreatic adenocarcinoma. Ann Surg Oncol 2011;18(3):636–41.
20. Jenkinson AD, Lim J, Agrawal N, et al. Laparoscopic feeding jejunostomy in esophagogastric cancer. Surg Endosc 2007;21(2):299–302.

21. Young MT, Troung H, Gebhart A, et al. Outcomes of laparoscopic feeding jejunostomy tube placement in 299 patients. Surg Endosc 2016;30(1):126–31.
22. Siow SL, Mahendran HA, Wong CM, et al. Laparoscopic T-tube feeding jejunostomy as an adjunct to staging laparoscopy for upper gastrointestinal malignancies: the technique and review of outcomes. BMC Surg 2017;17(1):25.
23. Watt AM, Faragher IG, Griffin TT, et al. Self-expanding metallic stents for relieving malignant colorectal obstruction: a systematic review. Ann Surg 2007;246(1):24–30.
24. Bohn KA, Ray CE. Repeat large-volume paracentesis versus tunneled peritoneal catheter placement for malignant ascites: a cost-minimization study. AJR Am J Roentgenol 2015;205(5):1126–34.
25. Valle SJ, Alzahrani NA, Alzahrani SE, et al. Laparoscopic hyperthermic intraperitoneal chemotherapy (HIPEC) for refractory malignant ascites in patients unsuitable for cytoreductive surgery. Int J Surg 2015;23(Pt A):176–80.
26. Ba M-C, Long H, Zhang X-L, et al. Laparoscopic hyperthermic intraperitoneal perfusion chemotherapy for patients with malignant ascites secondary to unresectable gastric cancer. J Laparoendosc Adv Surg Tech A 2016;26(1):32–9.
27. de Mestier L, Volet J, Scaglia E, et al. Is palliative laparoscopic hyperthermic intraperitoneal chemotherapy effective in patients with malignant hemorrhagic ascites? Case Rep Gastroenterol 2012;6(1):166–70.
28. Elias AW, Kasi PM, Stauffer JA, et al. The feasibility and safety of surgery in patients receiving immune checkpoint inhibitors: a retrospective Study. Front Oncol 2017;7:121.
29. Lens M, Bataille V, Krivokapic Z. Melanoma of the small intestine. Lancet Oncol 2009;10(5):516–21.
30. Dresler CM, Olak J, Herndon JE, et al. Phase III intergroup study of talc poudrage vs talc slurry sclerosis for malignant pleural effusion. Chest 2005;127(3):909–15.
31. Warren WH, Kim AW, Liptay MJ. Identification of clinical factors predicting Pleurx catheter removal in patients treated for malignant pleural effusion. Eur J Cardiothorac Surg 2008;33(1):89–94.
32. Fahy B. Fellowship training in hospice and palliative care: new pathways for surgeons. 2015. Available at: http://www.mdedge.com/acssurgerynews/article/101238/hospice-palliative-medicine/fellowship-training-hospice-and-palliative. Accessed December 18, 2017.

Robotic Developments in Cancer Surgery

Carolijn L.M.A. Nota, BSc[a,b,1,2], Francina Jasmijn Smits, MD[b,1,2],
Yanghee Woo, MD[a], Inne H.M. Borel Rinkes, MD, PhD[b,1],
Izaak Quintus Molenaar, MD, PhD[b,1], Jeroen Hagendoorn, MD, PhD[b,1],
Yuman Fong, MD[a,*]

KEYWORDS

• Robotics • Minimally invasive surgery • Oncologic surgery

KEY POINTS

• Robotic surgery is safe and feasible for a wide variety of procedures.
• Robotic surgery is being increasingly used in complex abdominal procedures.
• The use of robotics potentially extends indications for several procedures beyond what is possible with conventional laparoscopy but will not fully replace laparoscopy.

INTRODUCTION

Over the past few decades, cancer surgery has become more specialized and a wide variety of subdisciplines have been formed. Centralization of complex oncologic procedures, together with expanding indications, have led to increased volume of procedures in specialized centers, creating opportunities for innovation, such as the use of robotic technology in complex abdominal cancer surgeries.

In 2000 the US Food and Drug Administration approved the da Vinci surgical robot from Intuitive (Intuitive Surgical Inc, Sunnyvale, CA, USA) for the US market. The device was, among others, inspired by the call for telesurgical machines for President Dwight Eisenhower's Defense Advanced Research Projects Agency (DARPA). DARPA intended to develop remote surgery technology to treat wounded soldiers in war

Disclosure Statement: C.L.M.A. Nota, F.J. Smits, I.H.M. Borel Rinkes, I.Q. Molenaar, and J. Hagendoorn have declared no conflict of interest. Y. Fong is a scientific consultant to Medtronics Inc. Y. Woo is a scientific consultant to Johnson and Johnson Inc.
[a] Department of Surgery, City of Hope National Medical Center, 1500 East Duarte Road, Duarte, CA 91010, USA; [b] Department of Surgery, UMC Utrecht Cancer Center, University Medical Center Utrecht, Heidelberglaan 100, 3584 CX Utrecht, Netherlands
[1] Present address: Postbus 85500, 3508 GA, Utrecht, The Netherlands.
[2] Authors Carolijn L.M.A. Nota and Francina Jasmijn Smits have contributed equally to this work.
* Corresponding author.
E-mail address: yfong@coh.org

zones from a distance with telesurgery.[1] Intuitive Surgical Inc, seized the opportunity for the civilian market, bought the patents, and subsequently developed the first generation of da Vinci surgical robots.

For the first robots developed to assist in surgery one should go a bit further back in time. In 1984, the first experimental orthopedic surgeries using the Arthrobot were performed at the University of British Columbia. In the following years, several other robotic systems were developed for specific procedures, including PROBOT (purposed for prostatectomies), ROBODOC (purposed for hip replacements), and ZEUS by Computer Motion Inc, (purposed for microsurgery procedures in cardiac surgery). Computer Motion Inc, performed the first transatlantic robotic surgery, thereby fulfilling the promise of remote telesurgery. In 2001, surgeons in the United States performed a robotic cholecystectomy on a patient in Strasbourg, France. The procedure was completed in 54 minutes and the patient recovered without any complications.[2-7]

Entry of the da Vinci surgical robot in 2000 onto the market completely changed the field of minimally invasive surgery. The da Vinci surgical robot was initially approved for general surgery, but not long after its entrance on the market it found its way into minimally invasive surgery in many specialties. Over the past 18 years, the surgical robot was further developed and indications rapidly expanded. Even highly complex oncologic surgeries such as esophageal gastrectomies and liver and pancreatic resections are currently performed using the robot.[8-13] In this article, the authors discuss advances and technical developments in robotic surgery, with an emphasis on oncologic surgery.

CONVENTIONAL LAPAROSCOPY AND ROBOTIC SURGERY

Over the past few decades there has been increased utilization of minimally invasive surgery. Currently, conventional laparoscopy is the standard approach of treatment for several procedures, including cholecystectomy and appendectomy.[14-16] The benefits of minimally invasive surgery over open surgery include less blood loss, less postoperative pain, and quicker recovery from surgery and thus a shorter hospital stay.[17-19]

With the benefits of minimally invasive surgery being evident, surgeons have been exploring other, more advanced indications for conventional laparoscopic surgery. Hence, complex procedures such as Whipple procedures and extensive liver resections have been performed laparoscopically as well. However, the laparoscopic instruments have several technical limitations, which can be hindering when performing highly complex oncologic procedures. For example, instruments are straight and lack the ability to articulate, the technique requires the surgeon to move in opposite direction from what he is seeing on the screen, and the view on the operative field is usually 2-dimensional (2D). Moreover, ergonomics are poor.[20-22]

The robot was designed to overcome these restrictions. Robotic instruments are wristed and have a wider range of motion than the human hand, and motion scaling is standard set in a 1:3 ratio. The robot provides a magnified view of the operative field in 3D. Furthermore, ergonomics are optimized. Hence, a surgeon can perform minimally invasive surgery without compromising movement abilities and visibility. The disadvantages of the robotic technology include significantly increased costs.[20,23] Early in the robotic era, surgeons cited the lack of haptic feedback as a disadvantage. As more experience has been gained, a whole generation of surgeons has learned to operate at the highest level without reliance from haptic feedback.

Despite the aforementioned disadvantages, the robot currently is used in a wide variety of (oncologic) procedures. A retrospective study on the use of robotics across different specialties between 2008 and 2013 in the United States demonstrated that the proportion of procedures performed robotically doubled over the study period, increasing from 6.8% to 17%.[24] This increased interest in the use of minimally invasive surgery is also reflected on in research. Several randomized controlled trials are being executed comparing minimally invasive approaches (including conventional laparoscopy and robot-assisted laparoscopy) with open approaches.[25–27] There is no doubt that robotics has become an easy portal for entry into the minimally invasive surgical realm.

TECHNICAL ADVANCES OF ROBOTICS IN CANCER SURGERY

With extending indications and the fact that more and more complex oncologic surgeries are performed robotically nowadays, the current robotic systems are better equipped than the first generation brought to the market 17 years ago, with many new tools aimed at optimizing oncologic surgery.

The articulating instruments and a 3D, magnified view allow the surgeon to perform precise dissection with optimal dexterity. In addition, the most advanced surgical robot currently available is designed to allow multiquadrant surgery and its design prevents the robotic arms from colliding into each other.[20,28]

When operating with the robot, several technical innovations are available specifically for oncologic purposes. Among others, Firefly Fluorescence imaging has been developed. This technique uses near infrared technology to provide real-time imaging of anatomic structures. Indocyanine dye is administered to the patient and subsequently binds to albumin. A laser is used to visualize the dye. Using Firefly, blood vessels and bile ducts can be identified as well as malignancies. In the liver, because indocyanine green is metabolized by hepatocytes, the liver turns green while tumor tissues stay black. Using Firefly imaging, following a resection line along green fluorescent tissue ensures a negative margin (**Fig. 1**).[29] This is just the first optical tool of many being developed that will enhance safer and more effective cancer surgery. In the future, nerves, lymphatics, and metastatic tumors are likely to be visualized on the robotic console.

Other tools are available as well to provide optimal tumor visualization, such as robotic ultrasound and Tilepro technology multiscreen imaging. This allows up to 2 extra screens in the surgeon's field of view when sitting behind the console. Ultrasound images, computed tomography scans or any other imaging can be displayed next to the view of the operative field to help with tumor localization or for any other desired

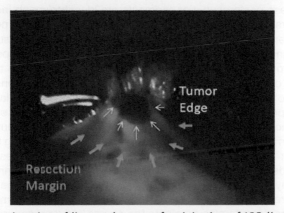

Fig. 1. Fluorescent imaging of liver and tumor after injection of ICG (*indocyanine green*). Liver is green and tumor stays black. Dissection in green area allows for confirmation of a negative margin. (*Courtesy of* Intuitive Surgical, Inc, Sunnyvale, CA.)

purpose. Using this technique, surgical efficiency can be increased as well.[30,31] It is likely that 3D reconstructions of preoperative cross-sectional imaging and biological imaging will be overlaid onto the optical images for guidance and navigation.

However, despite all the aforementioned technical tools available, the robot still has some technical disadvantages, from which some can be limiting in cancer surgery, foremost the lack of haptic feedback. Although several techniques are present for tumor visualization and localization, it's not (yet) possible to use the sense of touch when performing robotic surgery and thus feel a tumor. Hence, concerns have been expressed about the ability to obtain negative margins in robotic surgery. Most experienced robotic surgeons, however, have grown up in the field without reliance on haptic feedback. However, most surgeons would not seek haptic feedback; if implemented it will significantly increase cost or ruin the steady, precise feel without haptics.

ROBOTIC OUTCOMES IN KEY COMPLEX ABDOMINAL CANCER SURGERY

Several complex procedures in abdominal cancer surgery can specifically be identified, which, in theory, benefit the most from a robotic approach. For example, the optimized view and increased robotic dexterity are beneficial when constructing anastomoses in esophageal resection or in pancreatoduodenectomy or when performing extensive lymphadenectomy in a patient with gastric cancer. Moreover, the articulating robotic instruments allow for minimally invasive surgery in areas that are difficult to reach using conventional laparoscopy, including posterosuperior segment liver resection and total mesorectal excision for colorectal cancer. A few of these procedures are discussed in further detail later.

Liver Resections

Recently, the first randomized controlled trial comparing open and laparoscopic liver resections for colorectal liver metastases was published.[17] The laparoscopic approach was associated with several benefits over the open approach, including fewer complications and shorter hospital stay. However, in minor liver resections of the posterosuperior segments (ie, <4 segments including I, IVa, VII, and VIII), the anatomy makes these segments difficult to reach with conventional laparoscopic instrumentation.[32] In several studies on conventional laparoscopic liver resection, resections of these posterosuperior segments are identified as an independent predictor for conversion.[33,34] Hence, most of these resections are still performed open. In contrast, the articulating instruments of the robot are eminently suited for curved parenchymal transection, as needed in resection of the posterosuperior segments. A small number of studies reporting on robotic liver resections have been published, with acceptable outcomes in terms of complications and conversions. Outcomes of these studies are summarized in **Table 1**. The introduction of robotic surgery in liver resection could potentially extend indications for minimally invasive surgery.

Hepatic robotic surgery provides a good illustration as to the evolution of the field. The initial papers on robotic liver resections were on surgeons trying to do what they did in open liver surgery, only now using robotic techniques. These studies were instrumental in demonstrating feasibility of performing major surgery using robotic assistance. Many in the field have realized that the main advantage of robotic surgery is minimalization of skin and fascial trauma. The outcomes of major operations such as right trisectorectomies dominate the course of liver regeneration. However, the recovery of minor liver resections of tumors in poorly placed position are related to the fascial incision. In recent studies of robotic resections of poorly placed tumors,

Table 1
Summary outcomes on robotic liver resection

Authors	Robotic Liver Resections, No.	Blood Loss, mL	Conversions, No.	Patients with More than 1 Complication, No.	Length of Stay, Days	Mortality, No.
Giulianotti et al,[35] 2011	70	260 (20–2000)[b]	4	15	7 (2–26)[b]	0
Tsung et al,[36] 2014	57	200 (30–3600)[b]	4	11	4 (1–31)[b]	0
Wu et al,[37] 2014	38	325 ± 480[a]	2	3	8 ± 5[a]	0
Lai et al,[38] 2013	41	415 (10–3500)[b]	2	3	6 ± 4[a]	0
Troisi et al,[39] 2013	40	330 ± 300[a]	8	5	6 ± 3[a]	0
Choi et al,[40] 2012	30	345 (95–1500)[c]	2	13	12 (5–46)[b]	0
Spampinato et al,[41] 2014	25	250 (100–1900)[b]	1	4	8 (4–22)[b]	0
Felli et al,[42] 2015	20	50 (0–200)[c]	0	2	6 (4–14)[b]	0
Ji et al,[43] 2011	13	280[e]	0	1	7[e]	NR
Yu et al,[44] 2014	13	390 ± 65[a]	0	0	8 ± 2[a]	0
Berber et al,[45] 2010	9	135 ± 60[d]	1	1	NR	NR
Kandil et al,[46] 2013	7	100 (10–200)[c]	0	2	2 (1–5)[b]	0

Abbreviation: NR, not reported.
[a] Reported as mean ± SD.
[b] Reported as median (range).
[c] Reported as mean (range).
[d] Reported as mean ± SEM.
[e] Reported as mean

Adapted from Nota CL, Rinkes IHB, Molenaar IQ, et al. Robot-assisted laparoscopic liver resection: a systematic review and pooled analysis of minor and major hepatectomies. HPB (Oxford) 2016;18(2):115; with permission.

investigators report same day discharge for most patients[32] and early recovery of function.[47] Robotic surgery has converted hepatectomies to outpatient procedures.

Gastrectomy

In patients undergoing gastrectomy for gastric adenocarcinoma, the robotic platform offers several essential advantages over the conventional laparoscopic approach. The wristed instruments and magnified view of the operative field allow for a precise lymph node dissection, as needed in gastric cancer surgery. These technical enhancements of the robotic platform could result in higher number of harvested lymph nodes than open surgery. Recent meta-analysis comparing conventional laparoscopy with robotic surgery showed a reduction in blood loss in favor of the robotic approach, with no difference in number of harvested lymph nodes shown.[48] Thus, robotic approach is at least equivalent to the proven laparoscopic approach. In addition, long-term oncologic outcomes of laparoscopic approach and robotic approach are comparable.[49] Studies comparing robotic, open, and laparoscopic approaches in gastrectomy are summarized in **Table 2**.

Pancreatic Resection

Highly complex procedures such as pancreatic resection are increasingly performed minimally invasively as well. A systematic review and meta-analysis on open versus minimally invasive pancreatoduodenectomy showed shorter hospital stay and reduced blood loss in favor of the minimally invasive approach.[54] The articulating robotic instruments enable optimal surgical dexterity as needed during construction of the anastomoses in pancreatoduodenectomy. A retrospective study on robotic versus open pancreatoduodenectomy in 8 American expert centers showed a reduction in major complications and blood loss in robotic pancreatoduodenectomy compared with the open approach, although the robotic approach was associated with a longer operative time.[9] An overview of the outcomes of the 2 largest series ($\geq$200 procedures) on robotic pancreatic resection is provided in **Table 3**.

Despite the fact that robotic technology offers some advantages over conventional laparoscopy in certain procedures, it might not be best suited for the entire spectrum of minimally invasive surgeries. In some relatively "simple" procedures the technical advantages of the robotic technology might not be as outspoken to justify the higher costs and increased operative time.[56,57]

FUTURE DIRECTIONS

Several surgical robots from other companies are expected to be launched in the upcoming years, including machines from companies such as Verb Surgical (Verb Surgical Inc, Mountain View, CA, USA), Ethicon and Google's collaborative company, and Medtronic (Medtronic, Dublin, Ireland). These new entries into the robotic field are likely to bring down the costs associated with the robotic technology and push for further innovation.

Moreover, new machines might come with new interfaces, additional tools, and new techniques that have not been explored yet. For example, Auris Surgical (Redwood City, CA, USA) is set to launch a catheter robot that will assist in image-guided bronchoscopy. This is likely to revolutionize transbronchial therapies. In the future, advanced techniques such as image fusion and fully automated robotic systems will probably take on a bigger role. It will be interesting to see how a company like Google will incorporate its expertise in data processing in a new generation of surgical robots.

Table 2
Studies comparing robotic, laparoscopic, and open approaches to gastrectomy

Author and Year	Approach	No. of Patients	D2 Lymphadenectomy (%)	No. Lymph Nodes Harvested	EBL (mL)	Op Time (min)	Morbidity (%)	LOS (days)	Mortality (%)
Parisi et al,[50] 2017	Robotic	151	95	28 ± 11[a]	118 ± 68[a]	365 ± 81[a]	18	9 ± 6[a]	NR
	Lap.	151	95	25 ± 14[a]	96 ± 119[a]	220 ± 92[a]	12	9 ± 9[a]	NR
	Open	302	97	26 ± 12[a]	127 ± 80[a]	199 ± 60[a]	20	13 ± 6[a]	NR
Huang et al,[51] 2012	Robotic	39	87	32 ± 14[a]	50[b]	430[a]	15	7[b]	3
	Lap.	64	19	26 ± 12[a]	100[b]	350[a]	16	11[b]	2
	Open	586	88	34 ± 15[a]	400[b]	320[a]	15	12[b]	1
Kim et al,[52] 2012	Robotic	436	NR	40 ± 16[a]	85 ± 160[a]	226 ± 54	10	8 ± 14[a]	0.5
	Lap.	861	NR	38 ± 14[a]	112 ± 229[a]	176 ± 63	9	8 ± 9[a]	0.3
	Open	4542	NR	41 ± 17[a]	192 ± 193[a]	158 ± 52	11	10 ± 9[a]	0.5
Kim et al,[53] 2010	Robotic	16	88	41 ± 11[a]	30 ± 15[a]	259 ± 39[a]	0	5 ± 0.3	0
	Lap.	11	73	37 ± 10[a]	45 ± 37[a]	204 ± 36[a]	9	7 ± 1	0
	Open	12	100	43 ± 10[a]	79 ± 74[a]	127 ± 24[a]	17	7 ± 1	0

Abbreviations: EBL, estimated blood loss; NR, not reported.
[a] Reported as mean ± SD.
[b] Reported as median.

Table 3
Summary of the outcomes of the 2 largest case series on robotic pancreatic resection

Author	Patients (No.)	Estimated Blood Loss (mL)[a]	Conversion (No.)	Morbidity[b]	Length of Stay (days)	90-d Mortality (No.)
Zureikat et al,[10] 2013						
PD	132	300 (IQR: 150–600)	11	28	10 (4-87)[c]	5
DP	83	150 (IQR: 100–300)	2	11	6 (4–12)[c]	0
Central pancreatectomy	13	200 (IQR: 50–300)	2	3	8 (6–19)[c]	0
Enucleation	10	50 (IQR: 25–100)	0	3	5 (3–12)[c]	0
Total pancreatectomy	5	1000 (IQR: 400–1500)	1	1	10 (7–18)[c]	0
Appleby resection	5	200 (IQR: 200–400)	0	4	9 (6–14)[c]	0
Frey resection	4	100 (IQR: 75–150)	0	1	6 (5–9)[c]	0
Boggi et al,[55] 2016						
PD	83	NR	2	13	17 (14–26)[d]	2
DP	83	NR	1	2	10.0 (8.5–15)[d]	0
Central pancreatectomy	5	NR	0	0	17.5 (11.8–22)[d]	0
Enucleation	12	NR	0	0	7.0 (5.3–9.8)[d]	0
Total pancreatectomy	17	NR	0	2	23 (14.5–29.5)[d]	0

Abbreviations: DP, distal pancreatectomy; NR, not reported; PD, pancreatoduodenectomy.
[a] Reported as median (IQR).
[b] All Clavien-Dindo Grade III or IV complications.
[c] Reported as days (range).
[d] Reported as median (IQR).

In contrast, not only the market for surgical robots is changing, new conventional laparoscopic instruments are being developed as well, potentially with new features such as wristed instruments. The authors speculate that robotic surgery and conventional laparoscopy in their current forms will come closer together in the next few decades. However, it is believed that articulating instruments and 3D view are the future, in any form possible.

SUMMARY

Robotic surgery has experienced an extensive growth over the past 2 decades. Many studies in different fields of surgical oncology have displayed safety and feasibility of the robotic platform and comparable outcomes with conventional laparoscopy. In contrast to 20 years ago, complex procedures are performed using robotics nowadays and several technical tools, including Firefly technology and Tilepro multiscreen imaging, have become available to optimally facilitate oncologic surgery. Potentially, the use of robotics expands indications beyond what is possible using conventional laparoscopy, although it should be noted that the technology might not be best suited for the entire spectrum of minimally invasive surgeries.

REFERENCES

1. Bowersox JC, Cordts PR, LaPorta AJ. Use of an intuitive telemanipulator system for remote trauma surgery: an experimental study. J Am Coll Surg 1998;186(6): 615–21.
2. Hockstein NG, Gourin CG, Faust RA, et al. A history of robots: from science fiction to surgical robotics. J Robot Surg 2007;1(2):113–8.
3. Hussain A, Malik A, Halim MU, et al. The use of robotics in surgery: a review. Int J Clin Pract 2014;68(11):1376–82.
4. Leal Ghezzi T, Campos Corleta O. 30 Years of Robotic Surgery. World J Surg 2016;40(10):2550–7.
5. Surgical I. History of intuitive surgical. 2017. Available at: https://www.intuitivesurgical.com/company/history/. Accessed November 26, 2017.
6. Fong Y, Woo Y, Giulianotti PC. Robotic surgery: the promise and finally the progress. Hepatobiliary Surg Nutr 2017;6(4):219–21.
7. Marescaux J, Leroy J, Rubino F, et al. Transcontinental robot-assisted remote telesurgery: feasibility and potential applications. Ann Surg 2002;235(4):487–92.
8. Magge D, Zureikat A, Hogg M, et al. Minimally invasive approaches to pancreatic surgery. Surg Oncol Clin N Am 2016;25(2):273–86.
9. Zureikat AH, Postlewait LM, Liu Y, et al. A multi-institutional comparison of perioperative outcomes of robotic and open pancreaticoduodenectomy. Ann Surg 2016;264(4):640–9.
10. Zureikat AH, Moser AJ, Boone BA, et al. 250 robotic pancreatic resections: safety and feasibility. Ann Surg 2013;258(4):554–9 [discussion: 559–62].
11. Nota CL, Rinkes IHB, Molenaar IQ, et al. Robot-assisted laparoscopic liver resection: a systematic review and pooled analysis of minor and major hepatectomies. HPB (Oxford) 2016;18(2):113–20.
12. Woo Y, Hyung WJ, Pak KH, et al. Robotic gastrectomy as an oncologically sound alternative to laparoscopic resections for the treatment of early-stage gastric cancers. Arch Surg 2011;146(9):1086–92.
13. Ruurda JP, van der Sluis PC, van der Horst S, et al. Robot-assisted minimally invasive esophagectomy for esophageal cancer: a systematic review. J Surg Oncol 2015;112(3):257–65.

14. Lo CM, Liu CL, Lai EC, et al. Early versus delayed laparoscopic cholecystectomy for treatment of acute cholecystitis. Ann Surg 1996;223(1):37–42.
15. Bass EB, Pitt HA, Lillemoe KD. Cost-effectiveness of laparoscopic cholecystectomy versus open cholecystectomy. Am J Surg 1993;165(4):466–71.
16. Sohn M, Agha A, Bremer S, et al. Surgical management of acute appendicitis in adults: a review of current techniques. Int J Surg 2017;48:232–9.
17. Fretland AA, Dagenborg VJ, Bjornelv GMW, et al. Laparoscopic versus open resection for colorectal liver metastases: the OSLO-COMET randomized controlled trial. Ann Surg 2018;267(2):199–207.
18. Venkat R, Edil BH, Schulick RD, et al. Laparoscopic distal pancreatectomy is associated with significantly less overall morbidity compared to the open technique: a systematic review and meta-analysis. Ann Surg 2012;255(6):1048–59.
19. Kelly KJ, Selby L, Chou JF, et al. Laparoscopic versus open gastrectomy for gastric adenocarcinoma in the west: a case-control study. Ann Surg Oncol 2015;22(11):3590–6.
20. Leung U, Fong Y. Robotic liver surgery. Hepatobiliary Surg Nutr 2014;3(5): 288–94.
21. Ishizawa T, Gumbs AA, Kokudo N, et al. Laparoscopic segmentectomy of the liver: from segment I to VIII. Ann Surg 2012;256(6):959–64.
22. Sharpe SM, Talamonti MS, Wang CE, et al. Early national experience with laparoscopic pancreaticoduodenectomy for ductal adenocarcinoma: a comparison of laparoscopic pancreaticoduodenectomy and open pancreaticoduodenectomy from the national cancer data base. J Am Coll Surg 2015;221(1):175–84.
23. Barbash GI, Glied SA. New technology and health care costs–the case of robot-assisted surgery. N Engl J Med 2010;363(8):701–4.
24. Juo YY, Mantha A, Abiri A, et al. Diffusion of robotic-assisted laparoscopic technology across specialties: a national study from 2008 to 2013. Surg Endosc 2018; 32(3):1405–13.
25. van der Sluis PC, Ruurda JP, van der Horst S, et al. Robot-assisted minimally invasive thoraco-laparoscopic esophagectomy versus open transthoracic esophagectomy for resectable esophageal cancer, a randomized controlled trial (ROBOT trial). Trials 2012;13:230.
26. de Rooij T, van Hilst J, Vogel JA, et al. Minimally invasive versus open distal pancreatectomy (LEOPARD): study protocol for a randomized controlled trial. Trials 2017;18(1):166.
27. Haverkamp L, Brenkman HJ, Seesing MF, et al. Laparoscopic versus open gastrectomy for gastric cancer, a multicenter prospectively randomized controlled trial (LOGICA-trial). BMC Cancer 2015;15:556.
28. Yuh B, Yu X, Raytis J, et al. Use of a mobile tower-based robot—The initial Xi robot experience in surgical oncology. J Surg Oncol 2016;113(1):5–7.
29. Surgical I. Crystal clear 3D HD vision. 2017. Available at: https://intuitivesurgical.com/products/da-vinci-xi/3D-HD-vision.php. Accessed November 27, 2017.
30. Woo Y, Choi GH, Min BS, et al. Novel application of simultaneous multi-image display during complex robotic abdominal procedures. BMC Surg 2014;14:13.
31. Surgical I. da Vinci Si Extended Features. 2017. Available at: https://www.intuitivesurgical.com/products/davinci_surgical_system/davinci_surgical_system_si/features-benefits.php. Accessed November 27, 2017.
32. Melstrom LG, Warner SG, Woo Y, et al. Selecting incision-dominant cases for robotic liver resection: towards outpatient hepatectomy with rapid recovery. Hepatobiliary Surg Nutr 2018;7(2):77–84.

33. Halls MC, Cipriani F, Berardi G, et al. Conversion for unfavorable intraoperative events results in significantly worst outcomes during laparoscopic liver resection: lessons learned from a multicenter review of 2861 cases. Ann Surg 2017. https://doi.org/10.1097/SLA.0000000000002332.
34. Troisi RI, Montalti R, Van Limmen JG, et al. Risk factors and management of conversions to an open approach in laparoscopic liver resection: analysis of 265 consecutive cases. HPB (Oxford) 2014;16(1):75–82.
35. Giulianotti PC, Coratti A, Sbrana F, et al. Robotic liver surgery: results for 70 resections. Surgery 2011;149(1):29–39.
36. Tsung A, Geller DA, Sukato DC, et al. Robotic versus laparoscopic hepatectomy: a matched comparison. Ann Surg 2014;259(3):549–55.
37. Wu YM, Hu RH, Lai HS, et al. Robotic-assisted minimally invasive liver resection. Asian J Surg 2014;37(2):53–7.
38. Lai EC, Yang GP, Tang CN. Robot-assisted laparoscopic liver resection for hepatocellular carcinoma: short-term outcome. Am J Surg 2013;205(6):697–702.
39. Troisi RI, Patriti A, Montalti R, et al. Robot assistance in liver surgery: a real advantage over a fully laparoscopic approach? Results of a comparative bi-institutional analysis. Int J Med Robot 2013;9(2):160–6.
40. Choi GH, Choi SH, Kim SH, et al. Robotic liver resection: technique and results of 30 consecutive procedures. Surg Endosc 2012;26(8):2247–58.
41. Spampinato MG, Coratti A, Bianco L, et al. Perioperative outcomes of laparoscopic and robot-assisted major hepatectomies: an Italian multi-institutional comparative study. Surg Endosc 2014;28(10):2973–9.
42. Felli E, Santoro R, Colasanti M, et al. Robotic liver surgery: preliminary experience in a tertiary hepato-biliary unit. Updates Surg 2015;67(1):27–32.
43. Ji WB, Wang HG, Zhao ZM, et al. Robotic-assisted laparoscopic anatomic hepatectomy in China: initial experience. Ann Surg 2011;253(2):342–8.
44. Yu YD, Kim KH, Jung DH, et al. Robotic versus laparoscopic liver resection: a comparative study from a single center. Langenbecks Arch Surg 2014;399(8):1039–45.
45. Berber E, Akyildiz HY, Aucejo F, et al. Robotic versus laparoscopic resection of liver tumours. HPB (Oxford) 2010;12(8):583–6.
46. Kandil E, Noureldine SI, Saggi B, et al. Robotic liver resection: initial experience with three-arm robotic and single-port robotic technique. JSLS 2013;17(1):56–62.
47. Sun V, Dumitra S, Ruel N, et al. Wireless monitoring program of patient-centered outcomes and recovery before and after major abdominal cancer surgery. JAMA Surg 2017;152(9):852–9.
48. Chen K, Pan Y, Zhang B, et al. Robotic versus laparoscopic Gastrectomy for gastric cancer: a systematic review and updated meta-analysis. BMC Surg 2017;17:93.
49. Pan JH, Zhou H, Zhao XX, et al. Long-term oncological outcomes in robotic gastrectomy versus laparoscopic gastrectomy for gastric cancer: a meta-analysis. Surg Endosc 2017;31(10):4244–51.
50. Parisi A, Reim D, Borghi F, et al. Minimally invasive surgery for gastric cancer: a comparison between robotic, laparoscopic and open surgery. World J Gastroenterol 2017;23(13):2376–84.
51. Huang KH, Lan YT, Fang WL, et al. Initial experience of robotic gastrectomy and comparison with open and laparoscopic gastrectomy for gastric cancer. J Gastrointest Surg 2012;16(7):1303–10.
52. Kim KM, An JY, Kim HI, et al. Major early complications following open, laparoscopic and robotic gastrectomy. Br J Surg 2012;99(12):1681–7.

53. Kim MC, Heo GU, Jung GJ. Robotic gastrectomy for gastric cancer: surgical techniques and clinical merits. Surg Endosc 2010;24(3):610–5.
54. de Rooij T, Lu MZ, Steen MW, et al. Minimally invasive versus open pancreatoduodenectomy: systematic review and meta-analysis of comparative cohort and registry studies. Ann Surg 2016;264(2):257–67.
55. Boggi U, Napoli N, Costa F, et al. Robotic-assisted pancreatic resections. World J Surg 2016;40(10):2497–506.
56. Park JS, Choi GS, Park SY, et al. Randomized clinical trial of robot-assisted versus standard laparoscopic right colectomy. Br J Surg 2012;99(9):1219–26.
57. Souche R, Herrero A, Bourel G, et al. Robotic versus laparoscopic distal pancreatectomy: a French prospective single-center experience and cost-effectiveness analysis. Surg Endosc 2018;32(8):3562–9.

Transluminal Cancer Surgery

Antonio M. Lacy, MD, PhD*, Fransisco Borja De Lacy, MD,
Silvia Valverde, MD

KEYWORDS

- Transluminal cancer surgery • Natural orifice endoluminal surgery
- Laparoscopic surgery • Peroral endoscopic myotomy • Transanal (ta TME)

KEY POINTS

- Although approaches like transgastric or transvaginal cholecystectomy have had limited diffusion in the surgical community, peroral endoscopic myotomy and transanal total mesorectal excision (TaTME) have become accepted by many surgeons.
- Device development and training are major barriers to a broader application of natural orifices endoluminal surgery.
- When appropriately trained surgeons select patients with rectal cancer well, similar outcomes compared with other minimally invasive or open approaches can be achieved with TaTME.
- TaTME without transabdominal minimally invasive assistance remains practiced by a few surgeons and is at risk for compromising the oncologic quality of rectal cancer surgery if not practiced appropriately.

EVOLUTION OF TRANSLUMINAL SURGERY

Surgical oncology has undergone a major revolution over the last few years. The fast-growing technological advancements have undeniably influenced the emergence of new surgical techniques. The progress has become especially evident in the development of less traumatic surgery, as surgery has moved beyond open surgery to minimally invasive approaches, such as laparoscopy, robotic, or natural orifice endoluminal surgery (NOTES).[1] The progress was driven by surgeons eager to develop new surgical techniques with less morbidity. The Minimal Invasive Surgery (MIS) less postoperative pain, complications, wound infections, and hernia formation; improved cosmesis; lower short-term cost; and optimal midterm and long-term surgical and oncologic outcomes. Surgical evolution has been favored to a large extent by surgical instrumentation development, such as the discovery of the first rigid endoscopes by Desormeaux in 1865, which later would evolve into the first fiber-optic

Disclosure Statement: Dr A.M. Lacy is a consultant for MEDTRONIC, OLYMPUS, TOUCHSTONE, CONMED CORPORATION, APPLIED MEDICAL and JOHNSON & JOHNSON.
Department of Gastrointestinal Surgery, ICMDM, IDIBAPS, CIBEREHD, AIS Channel, Hospital Clínic, Universitat de Barcelona, Villarroel 170, 08036 Barcelona, Spain
* Corresponding author.
E-mail address: alacy@clinic.cat

endoscopy in 1957.[2] The change of open cholecystectomy to a laparoscopic approach took about 100 years; but in recent decades the technical evolution accelerated astonishingly; it took only 20 years to move from laparoscopy to transluminal surgery, that is, the first transgastric cholecystectomy. The improvement in surgical technology that enabled total laparoscopic surgery, hand-assisted laparoscopy, single-port laparoscopy, would later become the basis for natural orifice surgery or transluminal surgery. This surgical approach may probably be the most opposite approach to open surgery and remains controversial today.

Transluminal surgery encompasses several surgical procedures in which an endoscope is introduced through natural orifices (mouth, vagina, urethra, anus) thereby achieving scarless surgery. Therefore, NOTES can be considered less invasive than other minimally invasive procedures, such as laparoscopy or robotic surgery.[3] The journey to NOTES began long before the endoscope was invented because vaginal hysterectomies, a natural orifice surgery, has existed since Greek times[4] and can be considered the original natural orifice transluminal surgery. Despite the practice of vaginal hysterectomy in Greek times, similar to the delay in the progression from laparoscopic to NOTES, it was not until the sixteenth century that vaginal hysterectomy was brought back by Berengario da Carpi of Bologna in 1507.[5] Procedures, such as transperineal rectosigmoidectomy performed by Mikulicz in 1889, can also be considered early precursors of modern transluminal surgery.[6] Both of these operations (vaginal hysterectomy and transperineal rectosigmoidectomy) have all of the fundamental elements of NOTES, except they were not endoscopic. In the nineteenth century, inventions, such as the open-tube system with kerosene lamp light and mirrors, rigid endoscopes, rigid telescopic instruments, and semiflexible instruments that could be angled 30°, led to the world of endoscopy. Later, laparoscopy followed, which was embraced by gastroenterologists and surgeons alike.[1]

Even if transluminal surgery has initially been led by gastroenterologists as their skill set grew with procedures, such as the transluminal endoscopic drainage of a pancreatic pseudocyst,[3] the minimally invasive surgical experience from laparoscopy also pushed the limits of what could be accomplished endoluminally. In 2004, Anthony Kalloo and colleagues[7] performed the first transgastric peritoneoscopy in a porcine model, marking the beginning of a new era of minimally invasive surgery. Next, Rao and Reddy[8] demonstrated the first human case of transgastric NOTES appendectomy (circa 2004); the first transgastric cholecystectomy in a human was performed by Jacques Marescaux and colleagues.[9]

Thereupon, the term NOTES was coined to describe this novel approach, and the Natural Orifice Surgery Consortium for Assessment and Research (NOSCAR) was founded.[10] This group encompassed the American Society of Gastroenterology and the Society of American Gastrointestinal and Endoscopic Surgeons, led by David Rattner and Robert Hawes. NOSCAR was created to assess the indications, safety, and efficacy as well as the ethical use of NOTES in humans.[11–13]

CURRENT EVIDENCE AND TECHNIQUES

NOTES was initially performed and validated in benign pathologic conditions, such as cholecystectomies and appendectomies. Different surgical accesses were evaluated that include transgastric, transvaginal, and transrectal approaches.[14,15] Procedures are considered distant target NOTES because a healthy visceral organ is violated to gain surgical access. Most of these procedures are performed with a transvaginal or transgastric route and use a hybrid, laparoscopic-assisted technique. On the other hand, direct target NOTES does not violate a healthy visceral organ to gain access to another organ, such as in peroral endoscopic myotomy (POEM),[16] transanal total mesorectal excision (TaTME),[17] and vaginal access minimally invasive surgery for NOTES hysterectomy.[18]

NOTES cholecystectomy may be the most prominent transluminal operations considering the high incidence of cholecystectomy in general and application of a challenging technique to a straightforward operation. Several studies comparing transgastric and transvaginal approaches to laparoscopy have been published and include series with up to 750 patients.[19,20] Reported outcomes are less postoperative pain, analgesic requirements, and no major complications but a higher conversion rate. Further, cultural sensitivities as a reason for the limited diffusion of the transvaginal approach have been reported. Recently, a randomized trial initiated by NOSCAR comparing laparoscopic versus transgastric versus transvaginal[21] corroborated the safety profile for transvaginal cholecystectomy with noninferior clinical results, superior cosmesis, and a transient reduction in discomfort. The transgastric arm was closed because of lack of enrollment. In light of these results, the author no longer considers the transvaginal approach to cholecystectomy experimental.

Achalasia is an important risk factor for the development of esophageal cancer with an approximate increased risk of 28% and 3.3% of patients developing cancer. POEM[16,22–24] is an evolving therapeutic modality for achalasia based on a NOTES procedure. When compared with the gold standard, laparoscopic Heller myotomy (LHM), some studies show no differences between POEM and LHM in reduction in standardized assessment of dysphagia (Eckhart score), postoperative pain scores and analgesic requirements, length of hospital stay, adverse events, and symptomatic gastroesophageal reflux/reflux esophagitis. However, POEM showed a significantly lower operative time.[23] In contrast, other studies found that the incidence of reflux disease seems to be significantly more frequent after POEM than after LHM with fundoplication.[24] Multicenter randomized trials need to be conducted in patients with treatment-naïve achalasia and those who failed treatment to further assess the efficacy and safety of POEM.

Based on the published literature on NOTES, several meta-analyses have been reported.[25] These publication demonstrate the important progress in NOTES over the last 5 years.[26] One of these meta-analyses includes 6 randomized trials and 21 nonrandomized trials with 2186 patients undergoing different hybrid NOTES operations. The results correspond with prior data, demonstrating less postoperative pain, similar complication rates, and a higher cosmetic satisfaction with NOTES compared with laparoscopy.

The 5-year progress report on NOTES[26] highlighted the limited diffusion of NOTES in the surgical community due to the limited availability of specialized instruments and the risk of NOTES-specific complications. The most prominent NOTES-specific risk is the trauma inflicted to a virgin organ that otherwise would have not been violated. Other NOTES-specific complications that have been reported in addition to[27–31] rectal wall injury, perforation of the bladder, and cecal injury requiring laparotomy are pelvic abscess formation after cholecystectomy, vaginal bleeding and infection, gastric fistulae with peritonitis, gallbladder impaction in the proximal esophagus during specimen retrieval, esophageal hematoma, and perforation. Therefore, surgeons pioneering these techniques emphasize the need for caution, for significant experience with minimally invasive techniques for surgeons attempting NOTES and specific training.

After benign conditions were treated using NOTES, NOTES moved on to treating malignant pathologic conditions. In 2009, transanal minimally invasive surgery (TAMIS) took the lead using a transrectal approach to treat malignancy. TAMIS was developed as an alternative to conventional transanal local excision and transanal endoscopic microsurgery (TEM) for resection of rectal lesions, combining single-port access with the principles of transanal excision.[32] TEM was first conceived by Gerhard Buess[33] in 1983 as a platform that allowed removing benign lesions of the mid and upper rectum not easily accessible by conventional transanal methods. Since its first description, the use of TEM has proven to result in high-quality excisions with outcomes that are more favorable than standard transanal techniques for local excision because of a very low recurrence rate.[34–36] However, the advanced transanal platform requires specific instrumentation with associated high cost, ergonomic difficulties, and a steep learning curve.[35,37] For these reasons, TEM is primarily performed by a small number of high-volume specialists in referral centers; its adoption has been limited.[38]

The inception of TAMIS using single-port surgery devices was a solution to the high cost and the steep learning curve requiring specialized training to master TEM.[32,36,38] The availability of these platforms is due to its previous application to abdominal surgery and subsequent adoption for transanal use. Their lower cost compared with the specialized and expensive TEM equipment led to the increasing use of TAMIS. It enabled transanal endoscopic surgery to be performed at centers not equipped with a TEM platforms. Although TAMIS was initially performed in the United States, its utilization has rapidly spread worldwide because of its accessibility and the number of training courses available for surgeons. This increased utilization is reflected in the increasing number of publications since its inception in 2009.

Several small series and case reports have been published demonstrating TAMIS to be a feasible, low-cost alternative to TEM.[39–50] Indications for TAMIS rapidly moved from challenging to resect benign lesions only to histologically favorable early rectal cancers as well as palliative resections of cT2 or cT3 and ypT0 cancers.[36,38] Reports demonstrated that margin positivity and the tumor fragmentation rate improved when compared with Parks resection. The overall margin positivity has been reported to be between 7% and 10%, and the fragmentation rate lies between 5% and 7%.[38,40,45,48] The reported TAMIS operative time is lower than for TEM.[39,41,50] Postoperative morbidity has been recorded in 11% of patients. This morbidity includes hemorrhage (9%), urinary retention (4%), and scrotal or subcutaneous emphysema (3%) as the most common.[39] Local recurrence has been reported to be between 5% and 10%.[39,41,49] Therefore, local excision of appropriately selected patients with rectal neoplasia by TAMIS is a safe and feasible option with low morbidity and the advantage of organ preservation.

TAMIS development led to the next revolution in transluminal cancer surgery: transanal Total Mesorectal Excision (taTME), so-called NOTES TME or TaTME. TaTME has become the predominant technique of transluminal cancer surgery.[51–53] Its aim is to remove the rectum and the mesorectal envelope in patients with cancer. Its inception was motivated by the technical challenge of mid and low rectal cancer surgery via the standard transabdominal approach. These low-lying cancers that are difficult to access via a transabdominal approach occur typically in obese men with a narrow pelvis.[53,54] Although the advantages of TaTME is most evident in male patients with visceral obesity, a wide variety of patients with low rectal cancer benefit from this approach.[54]

TaTME is fundamentally a NOTES operation with laparoscopic assistance and is being increasingly performed by expert colorectal surgeons worldwide.[14] It combines 4 principal concepts and techniques: It merges TEM and TAMIS, which enables access to the rectum for the excision of benign and early cancer lesions and the transanal-transabdominal operation originally described by Gerald Marks and colleagues[55,56] for open surgery as the "down-to-up approach" for TME it also incorporates the TME technique itself, described by Bill Heald,[57] and applies it to a NOTES concept.

This transluminal technique was initially demonstrated in swine models with the goal of assessing the feasibility of the technique. This technique was pioneered by Patricia Sylla and colleagues[58] with laparoscopic instruments. In 2007, Mark Whiteford, Peter Denk, and Lee Swanström[59,60] reported their experience of 3 cases of the first total NOTES transanal rectosigmoidectomy using a TEM apparatus in a cadaveric model. Subsequently, Sylla and Lacy[61] performed the first NOTES transanal TME with laparoscopic assistance on a live patient.

Since these initial experiences with this technique, this approach was adopted by colorectal, oncologic, and minimally invasive surgeons worldwide. Early clinical series of transanal TME described the transanal approach for rectal cancer with laparoscopic assistance.[52,61–63] Outcomes showed adequate pathologic outcomes with negative distal and circumferential margins and intact specimens in all cases. The overall intraoperative and postoperative complication rates have been reported to be between 8.3% and 27.8%, respectively, which is similar to laparoscopic TME. Initial experiences emphasized the advantages of TaTME, which includes optimal visualization of the distal rectum and improved access to the distal pelvis. These initial studies demonstrate TaTME using laparoscopic guidance to be clinically feasible and safe when performed in carefully selected patients by surgeons with adequate surgical expertise and appropriate procedural training.[63]

The publication of larger series soon followed these initial case reports as experience increased in reference centers. These larger series report not only on the technical aspects but also morbidity and oncologic outcomes. Technical modifications of the initial approach followed,[53] which include the 2-team approach (the so-called Cecil approach) and the use of continuous flow insufflation and indocyanine green for vascular assessment. These technical modifications are a major step forward towards the standardization and the improvement of the technique. Two surgical teams working simultaneously have reduced the operative time and improved the feasibility, efficacy, and safety of the dissection. New-generation insufflators allow for a more constant pneumorectum, preventing rectal bellowing and allowing for efficient smoke evacuation. Vascular assessment with indocyanine green allows for the assessment of perfusion at the level of the anastomotic limbs with the goal of reducing anastomotic leaks.[64,65]

With these developments,[66–71] the mean operative time ranges from 166 to 315 minutes; morbidity ranges from 18% to 39%; macroscopic quality assessment of the resected specimen ranges from 88% to 98%; the local recurrence rate ranges from 0% to 2.3%; systemic recurrence rates range from 5.0% to 7.6%. Recent studies focusing on the histology results only[72] showed a complete mesorectal specimen in 95.7% of cases and a positive circumferential radial margin (CRM) (≤ 1 mm) and distal radial margin (DRM) (≤ 1 mm) rate of 8.1% and 3.2%, respectively. The optimal oncologic approach of complete mesorectal excision, negative CRM, and negative DRM was achieved in 88.1% (n = 155) of patients. These data contrast with the outcomes from a systematic review comparing the results of open versus laparoscopic rectal resections.[73] A meta-analysis included 14 unique randomized controlled trials with 2989 patients undergoing rectal resection. A noncomplete (nearly complete and incomplete) mesorectal excision was reported in 13.2% of laparoscopic cases with a rate of 10.4% in open cases. Positive CRM was found in 7.9% of laparoscopic and 6.1% of open cases. Since the reported data on specimen quality as a surrogate marker of oncologic quality and long-term survival lies within what has been reported for other minimally invasive and open approaches, TaTME performed by well-trained surgeons can be considered an appropriate technique to treat selected patients with rectal cancer.

Further, numerous smaller series and also meta-analyses have been published. For example, a meta-analysis[74] of 16 clinical studies included 150 patients undergoing TaTME. In all but 15 cases, transabdominal assistance was used. A positive circumferential resection margin was reported in 16 (11.8%) patients. Postoperative complications occurred in 34 (22.7%) patients.

However, data in the meta-analysis were not homogeneous and suggested the need for further quality control. Therefore, with the increase in the number of transanal surgeries performed, an international registry of TaTME patients was created to collect data from different institutions to precisely and transparently analyze outcomes of the technique. In a recent report, a total of 720 consecutively registered cases have been analyzed. This series included 634 patients with rectal cancer and 86 with benign conditions.[51] In this series, an intact TME specimen was achieved in 85% and postoperative mortality and morbidity were 0.5% and 32.6%, respectively. Risk factors for poor specimen quality (suboptimal TME specimen, perforation, and/or R1 resection) on multivariate analysis were a CRM at risk on preoperative staging MRI, low rectal tumor of less than 2 cm from the anorectal junction, and laparoscopic transabdominal posterior dissection to less than 4 cm from the anal verge. Five cases of urethral injury were described, which is a particularly concerning morbidity of this technique. The frequency of low ureteral injury has led experts to advice-specific training for TaTME to prevent morbidities, such as ureteral injury.

A later subanalysis of the anastomotic failure rate of the cases registered[75] revealed an overall anastomotic failure rate was 15.7%, which included early (7.8%) and delayed leak (2.0%), pelvic abscess (4.7%), anastomotic fistula (0.8%), chronic sinus (0.9%), and anastomotic stricture in 3.6% of cases. Independent risk factors of anastomotic failure were male sex, obesity, smoking, diabetes mellitus, tumors greater than 25 mm, excessive intraoperative blood loss, hand-sewn anastomosis, and prolonged perineal operative time. According to these results, large tumors in obese, diabetic male patients who smoke have the highest risk of anastomotic failure.

Studies have aimed at validating TaTME by comparing it with standard techniques. The group of Marks and colleagues[76] matched a cohort of 12 TMEs and 5 abdominoperineal resections to 2 cohorts operated on with different techniques: one cohort had the surgery performed transanally and the other one laparoscopically. The positive-circumferential margin rate was 0% versus 5.9% ($P = .32$); complete or near-complete TMEs were 100% versus 94.1% ($P = .32$); local recurrence was 5.9% versus 0% ($P = .32$). Xu and colleagues[77] reached the same conclusion when analyzing the data of 209 TaTME patients and 257 laproscopic total mesorectal excision (Lap TME) patients from 7 studies, which showed a wider CRM, lower rate of positive CRM, complete TME rate, and less operative time in favor of the TaTME, with no significant differences in the remainder of the analyzed parameters. Therefore, the data favored TaTME because a wider CRM, lower risk of positive CRM, higher complete TME rate, and shorter operative duration could be achieved.

Following these reports on the safety of TaTME with laparoscopic transabdominal assistance, Mark's group[78] followed the lead of Leroy and colleagues[79] and pushed the envelope farther by completing TaTME entirely transanally with no laparoscopic assistance. This experience suggests the feasibility and safety of a true NOTES TME and may be the future direction of this technique. Despite this development, this approach has not been widely adopted because of its technical difficulties. In order to ensure patient safety, TaTME without laparoscopic transabdominal assistance cannot be recommended today.

FUTURE OF TRANSLUMINAL SURGERY

Transluminal surgery is the most extreme form of the concept of minimally invasive surgery. In appropriately selected patients, it is a safe, effective, and scarless surgery performed through natural orifices. The benefits of transluminal surgery revolve around the decreased number and size of incisions resulting in improved cosmesis, less postoperative pain, less wound infections, and less hernias.

As Atallah and colleagues[14] pointed out, the diffusion and development of NOTES has increased over the last few years and resulted in greater clinical experience. However, there are ongoing challenges for NOTES, such as the limited ability to establish spatial orientation or to maintain a constant and safe insufflation pressure (within the peritoneal cavity), complications specific to transvisceral access (bacterial contamination of the peritoneal cavity), design limitations of available instrumentation, or lack of formal training programs for surgeons and endoscopists.

Industry's contribution is key for the wider implementation of NOTES and to overcome the technical difficulties surgeons face with NOTES.[80,81] The current endoscopic instrumentation is not specifically designed for intra-abdominal use and will require further development to make the pure NOTES approaches safer and more accessible. For example, straight and rigid laparoscopic instrumentation, especially when used for a single-access approach, hinders access to the entire abdominal cavity. However, once the technical limitations are overcome by technical developments from industry partners, more complex and novel procedures may be possible to be performed transluminally.

Early experiences with NOTES comprised essentially benign conditions. This experience would later lead to more complex procedures for malignant lesions, such as TME. Nowadays, POEM and TAMIS are the only pure NOTES surgeries that have established a place in the armamentarium of surgeons.[80] Other transluminal procedures are mostly performed in a hybrid fashion, such as TaTME itself.

TAMIS has become a well-established technique compared with other transanal platforms for local resection. The discussion is now centered around the optimal indications when this procedure is performed as part of a multimodal treatment concept that includes adjuvant therapy. Promising results are being published in favor of organ preservation techniques with adequate oncologic control.[82,83] Notwithstanding, multiple trials are ongoing, such as the transanal endoscopic microsurgery (TEM) and radiotherapy in early rectal cancer (TREC) and STAR-TREC trials,[84] which may expand the indications of this transluminal technique in patients with cancer.

TaTME is an excellent application of NOTES because it maintains the previously mentioned advantages of NOTES while allowing for excellent access to the distal rectum.[85,86] Although TaTME is not an entirely scarless surgery, it provides optimal surgical access for a technically highly demanding operation. In this context, it is reassuring that several studies have reported its safety and feasibility, with promisingly low morbidity and optimal oncologic results.

Today, structured training remains critical in reducing TaTME's specific morbidity, such as urethral injuries.[14,51,87,88] An international consensus conference[89,90] recommended standardized training programs that will flatten the learning curve and make this technique accessible for surgeons. In addition, randomized controlled trials are needed to assess NOTES in comparison with other approaches. This assessment will be performed in the future in the colon carcinoma laparoscopic or open resection (COLOR) III trial, which will compare TaTME to laparoscopic TME.[85] Additionally, trials comparing open versus laparoscopic versus robotic versus transanal approaches should be the next step to elucidate which technique is optimal for rectal surgery.

In conclusion, NOTES procedures are still being validated and require further developments in instrumentation to move procedures, such as TaTME, from a hybrid to a pure NOTES procedures. Benign condition have been an area that allowed for technical and procedural development so that the benefits of NOTES can now be applied to oncologic surgery. Nevertheless, given the complexity of NOTES, it is recommended to have NOTES and TaTME be performed by experienced surgeons only.

Rattner and Smith[80] and Hawes[81] pointed out, today NOTES is not meant to substitute laparoscopy but rather to complement laparoscopy and endoscopy, improving patient outcome requiring. To allow development in this field, a closer collaboration between surgeons and endoscopists is required.

REFERENCES

1. Rosin D. History in minimal access medicine and surgery. In: Rosin D, editor. Minimal Access Medicine and Surgery. Oxford (England): Radcliffe Medical Press; 1993. p. 1–9.

2. Lau WY, Leow CK, Li AK. History of endoscopic and laparoscopic surgery. World J Surg 1997;21(4):444–53.

3. Rattner D, Hawes RH. NOTES: gathering momentum. Surg Endosc 2006;20(5): 711–2.

4. Geller EJ. Vaginal hysterectomy: the original minimally invasive surgery. Minerva Ginecol 2014;66(1):23–33.

5. De Santo NG, Bisaccia C, De Santo LS, et al. Berengario da Carpi. Am J Nephrol 1999;19(2):199–212.

6. Mikulicz J. Zur operativen behandlung des prolapsus recti et coli invaginati. Arch Klin Chir 1889;38:74–97.

7. Kalloo AN, Singh VK, Jagannath SB, et al. Flexible transgastric peritoneoscopy: a novel approach to diagnostic and therapeutic interventions in the peritoneal cavity. Gastrointest Endosc 2004;60(1):114–7.

8. Reddy N, Rao P. Per oral transgastric endoscopic appendectomy in human. Proceedings of the 45th Annual Conference of the Society of Gastrointestinal Endoscopy of India. Jaipur, India, 28–29 February 2004.

9. Marescaux J, Dallemagne B, Perretta S, et al. Surgery without scars: report of transluminal cholecystectomy in a human being. Arch Surg 2007;142(9):823–6.

10. Hawes RH. Transition from laboratory to clinical practice in NOTES: role of NOSCAR. Gastrointest Endosc Clin N Am 2008;18(2):333–41.

11. Rattner D, Kalloo A, ASGE/SAGES Working Group. ASGE/SAGES Working Group on Natural Orifice Translumenal Endoscopic Surgery. October 2005. Surg Endosc 2006;20(2):329–33. No abstract available.

12. ASGE, SAGES. ASGE/SAGES Working Group on Natural Orifice Translumenal Endoscopic Surgery White Paper October 2005 [review]. Gastrointest Endosc 2006;63(2):199–203. No abstract available.

13. Rattner DW, SAGES/ASGE Joint Committee on NOTES. NOTES: where have we been and where are we going? Surg Endosc 2008;22(5):1143–5.

14. Atallah S, Martin-Perez B, Keller D, et al. Natural-orifice transluminal endoscopic surgery. Br J Surg 2015;102(2):e73–92.

15. Mohan HM, O'Riordan JM, Winter DC. Natural-orifice translumenal endoscopic surgery (NOTES): minimally invasive evolution or revolution? Surg Laparosc Endosc Percutan Tech 2013;23(3):244–50.

16. Khashab MA, Sharaiha RZ, Saxena P, et al. Novel technique of auto-tunneling during peroral endoscopic myotomy (with video). Gastrointest Endosc 2013; 77(1):119–22.

17. Lee GC, Sylla P. Shifting paradigms in minimally invasive surgery: applications of transanal natural orifice transluminal endoscopic surgery in colorectal surgery. Clin Colon Rectal Surg 2015;28(3):181–93.

18. Atallah S, Martin-Perez B, Albert M, et al. Vaginal access minimally invasive surgery (VAMIS): a new approach to hysterectomy. Surg Innov 2015;22(4):344–7.

19. Benhidjeb T, Kosmas IP, Hachem F, et al. Laparoscopic cholecystectomy versus transvaginal natural orifice transluminal endoscopic surgery cholecystectomy: results of a prospective comparative single-center study. Gastrointest Endosc 2018;87(2):509–16.

20. Peng C, Ling Y, Ma C, et al. Safety outcomes of NOTES cholecystectomy versus laparoscopic cholecystectomy: a systematic review and meta-analysis. Surg Laparosc Endosc Percutan Tech 2016;26(5):347–53.

21. Schwaitzberg SD, Roberts K, Romanelli JR, et al, Natural Orifice Surgery Consortium for Assessment and Research® (NOSCAR®) Clinical Trial Group. The NOVEL trial: natural orifice versus laparoscopic cholecystectomy-a prospective, randomized evaluation. Surg Endosc 2017. https://doi.org/10.1007/s00464-017-5955-5.

22. Stavropoulos SN, Desilets DJ, Fuchs KH, et al. Per-oral endoscopic myotomy white paper summary. Surg Endosc 2014;28(7):2005–19.

23. Talukdar R, Inoue H, Nageshwar Reddy D. Efficacy of peroral endoscopic myotomy (POEM) in the treatment of achalasia: a systematic review and meta-analysis. Surg Endosc 2015;29(11):3030–46.

24. Repici A, Fuccio L, Maselli R, et al. Gastroesophageal reflux disease after peroral endoscopic myotomy as compared with Heller's myotomy with fundoplication: a systematic review with meta-analysis. Gastrointest Endosc 2017. https://doi.org/10.1016/j.gie.2017.10.022.

25. Steinemann DC, Müller PC, Probst P, et al. Meta-analysis of hybrid natural-orifice transluminal endoscopic surgery versus laparoscopic surgery. Br J Surg 2017; 104(8):977–89.

26. Rattner DW, Hawes R, Schwaitzberg S, et al. The second SAGES/ASGE White Paper on natural orifice transluminal endoscopic surgery: 5 years of progress. Surg Endosc 2011;25(8):2441–8.

27. Arezzo A, Zornig C, Mofid H, et al. The EURO-NOTES clinical registry for natural orifice transluminal endoscopic surgery: a 2-year activity report. Surg Endosc 2013;27(9):3073–84.

28. Lehmann KS, Ritz JP, Wibmer A, et al. The German registry for natural orifice translumenal endoscopic surgery: report of the first 551 patients. Ann Surg 2010;252(2):263–70.

29. Zorron R, Palanivelu C, Galvão Neto MP, et al. International multicenter trial on clinical natural orifice surgery–NOTES IMTN study: preliminary results of 362 patients. Surg Innov 2010;17(2):142–58.

30. Wood SG, Panait L, Duffy AJ, et al. Complications of transvaginal natural orifice transluminal endoscopic surgery: a series of 102 patients. Ann Surg 2014;259(4): 744–9.

31. Mofid H, Emmermann A, Alm M, et al. Is the transvaginal route appropriate for intra-abdominal NOTES procedures? Experience and follow-up of 222 cases. Surg Endosc 2013;27(8):2807–12.

32. Atallah S, Albert M, Larach S. Transanal minimally invasive surgery: a giant leap forward. Surg Endosc 2010;24:2200–5.
33. Buess G, Hutterer F, Theiss J, et al. A system for a transanal endoscopic rectum operation. Chirurg 1984;55:677–80.
34. de Graaf EJ, Burger JW, van Ijsseldijk AL, et al. Transanal endoscopic microsurgery is superior to transanal excision of rectal adenomas. Colorectal Dis 2011;13: 762–7.
35. Middleton PF, Sutherland LM, Maddern GJ. Transanal endoscopic microsurgery: a systematic review. Dis Colon Rectum 2005;48:270–84.
36. Cataldo PA. Transanal endoscopic microsurgery. Surg Clin North Am 2006;86: 915–25.
37. Maya A, Vorenberg A, Oviedo M, et al. Learning curve for transanal endoscopic microsurgery: a single-center experience. Surg Endosc 2014;28(5):1407–12.
38. Rimonda R, Arezzo A, Arolfo S, et al. TransAnal minimally invasive surgery (TAMIS) with SILS Port versus Transanal Endoscopic Microsurgery (TEM): a comparative expermiental study. Surg Endosc 2013;27:3762–8.
39. Martin-Perez B, Andrade-Ribeiro GD, Hunter L, et al. A systematic review of transanal minimally invasive surgery (TAMIS) from 2010 to 2013 [review]. Tech Coloproctol 2014;18(9):775–88.
40. Albert MR, Atallah SB, deBeche-Adams TC, et al. Transanal minimally invasive surgery (TAMIS) for local excision of benign neoplasms and early-stage rectal cancer: efficacy and outcomes in the first 50 patients. Dis Colon Rectum 2013; 56(3):301–7.
41. Lee L, Burke JP, deBeche-Adams T, et al. Transanal minimally invasive surgery for local excision of benign and malignant rectal neoplasia: outcomes from 200 consecutive cases with midterm follow up. Ann Surg 2017. https://doi.org/10. 1097/SLA.0000000000002190.
42. Khoo RE. Transanal excision of a rectal adenoma using single access laparoscopic port. Dis Colon Rectum 2010;53:1078–9.
43. Ragupathi M, Haas EM. Transanal endoscopic video-assisted excision: application of single-port access. JSLS 2011;15:53–8.
44. van den Boezem PB, Kruyt PM, Stommel MW, et al. Transanal single-port surgery for the resection of large polyps. Dig Surg 2011;28(5–6):412–6.
45. Lim SB, Seo SI, Lee JL, et al. Feasibility of transanal minimally invasive surgery for mid-rectal lesions. Surg Endosc 2012;26(11):3127–32.
46. Hompes R, Ris F, Cunningham C, et al. Transanal glove port is a safe and cost-effective alternative for transanal endoscopic microsurgery. Br J Surg 2012; 99(10):1429–35.
47. McLemore EC, Coker A, Jacobsen G, et al. eTAMIS: endoscopic visualization for transanal minimally invasive surgery. Surg Endosc 2013;27(5):1842–5.
48. Barendse RM, Doornebosch PG, Bemelman WA, et al. Transanal employment of single access ports is feasible for rectal surgery. Ann Surg 2012;256(6):1030–3.
49. Lee L, Edwards K, Hunter IA, et al. Quality of local excision for rectal neoplasms using transanal endoscopic microsurgery versus transanal minimally invasive surgery: a multi-institutional matched analysis. Dis Colon Rectum 2017;60(9): 928–35.
50. Clancy C, Burke JP, Albert MR, et al. Transanal endoscopic microsurgery versus standard transanal excision for the removal of rectal neoplasms: a systematic review and meta-analysis [review]. Dis Colon Rectum 2015;58(2):254–61.

51. Penna M, Hompes R, Arnold S, et al, TaTME Registry Collaborative. Transanal total mesorectal excision: international registry results of the first 720 cases. Ann Surg 2017;266(1):111–7.
52. de Lacy AM, Rattner DW, Adelsdorfer C, et al. Transanal natural orifice transluminal endoscopic surgery (NOTES) rectal resection: "down-to-up" total mesorectal excision (TME)–short-term outcomes in the first 20 cases. Surg Endosc 2013; 27(9):3165–72.
53. Arroyave MC, DeLacy FB, Lacy AM. Transanal total mesorectal excision (TaTME) for rectal cancer: step by step description of the surgical technique for a two-teams approach. Eur J Surg Oncol 2017;43(2):502–5.
54. Heald RJ. A new solution to some old problems: transanal TME. Tech Coloproctol 2013;17(3):257–8.
55. Marks J, Mizrahi B, Dalane S, et al. Laparoscopic transanal abdominal transanal resection with sphincter preservation for rectal cancer in the distal 3 cm of the rectum after neoadjuvant therapy. Surg Endosc 2010;24(11):2700–7.
56. Marks J, Frenkel J, D'Andrea A, et al. Maximizing rectal cancer results: TEM and TATA techniques to expand sphincter preservation. J Surg Oncol 2011;20(3): 501–20.
57. Heald RJ. The 'Holy Plane' of rectal surgery. J R Soc Med 1988;81(9):503–8.
58. Sylla P, Willingham FF, Sohn DK, et al. NOTES rectosigmoid resection using transanal endoscopic microsurgery (TEM) with transgastricendoscopic assistance: a pilot study in swine. J Gastrointest Surg 2008;12(10):1717–23.
59. Whiteford MH, Denk PM, Swanström LL. Feasibility of radical sigmoid colectomy performed as natural orifice translumenal endoscopic surgery (NOTES) using transanal endoscopic microsurgery. Surg Endosc 2007;21(10):1870–4.
60. Denk PM, Swanström LL, Whiteford MH. Transanal endoscopic microsurgical platform for natural orifice surgery. Gastrointest Endosc 2008;68(5):954–9.
61. Sylla P, Rattner DW, Delgado S, et al. NOTES transanal rectal cancer resection using transanal endoscopic microsurgery and laparoscopic assistance. Surg Endosc 2010;24(5):1205–10.
62. Chouillard E, Chahine E, Khoury G, et al. NOTES total mesorectal excision (TME) for patients with rectal neoplasia: a preliminary experience. Surg Endosc 2014; 28(11):3150–7.
63. Einhoff IA, Lee GC, Sylla P. Transanal colorectal resection using natural orifice translumenal endoscopic surgery (NOTES). Dig Endosc 2014;26(Suppl 1):29–42.
64. Cassinotti E, Costa S, DE Pascale S, et al. How to reduce surgical complications in rectal cancer surgery using fluorescence techniques. Minerva Chir 2018;73(2): 210–6.
65. Keller DS, Ishizawa T, Cohen R, et al. Indocyanine green fluorescence imaging in colorectal surgery: overview, applications, and future directions. Lancet Gastroenterol Hepatol 2017;2(10):757–66.
66. Lacy AM, Tasende MM, Delgado S, et al. Transanal total mesorectal excision for rectal cancer: outcomes after 140 patients. J Am Coll Surg 2015;221(2):415–23.
67. Veltcamp Helbach M, Deijen CL, Velthuis S, et al. Transanal total mesorectal excision for rectal carcinoma: short-term outcomes and experience after 80 cases. Surg Endosc 2016;30(2):404–70.
68. Durke JP, Martin-Perez B, Khan A, et al. Transanal total mesorectal excision for rectal cancer: early outcomes in 50 consecutive patients. Colorectal Dis 2016; 18(6):570–7.
69. Buchs NC, Nicholson GA, Yeung T, et al. Transanal rectal resection: an initial experience of 20 cases. Colorectal Dis 2016;18(1):45–50.

70. Wolthuis AM, De Buck Van Overstraeten A, D'Hoore A. Laparoscopic NOSE colectomy with a camera sleeve: a technique in evolution. Colorectal Dis 2015; 17(5):O123–5.
71. Rouanet P, Mourregot A, Azar CC, et al. Transanal endoscopic proctectomy: an innovative procedure for difficult resection of rectal tumors in men with narrow pelvis. Dis Colon Rectum 2013;56(4):408–15.
72. de Lacy FB, van Laarhoven JJEM, Pena R, et al. Transanal total mesorectal excision: pathological results of 186 patients with mid and low rectal cancer. Surg Endosc 2017. https://doi.org/10.1007/s00464-017-5944-8.
73. Martínez-Pérez A, Carra MC, Brunetti F, et al. Pathologic outcomes of laparoscopic vs open mesorectal excision for rectal cancer: a systematic review and meta-analysis [review]. JAMA Surg 2017;152(4):e165665.
74. Araujo SE, Crawshaw B, Mendes CR, et al. Transanal total mesorectal excision: a systematic review of the experimental and clinical evidence. Tech Coloproctol 2015;19(2):69–82.
75. Penna M, Hompes R, Arnold S, et al, International TaTME Registry Collaborative. Incidence and risk factors for anastomotic failure in 1594 patients treated by transanal total mesorectal excision: results from the international TaTME registry. Ann Surg 2018. https://doi.org/10.1097/SLA.0000000000002653.
76. Marks JH, Montenegro GA, Salem JF, et al. Transanal TATA/TME: a case-matched study of taTME versus laparoscopic TME surgery for rectal cancer. Tech Coloproctol 2016;20(7):467–73.
77. Xu W, Xu Z, Cheng H, et al. Comparison of short-term clinical outcomes between transanal and laparoscopic total mesorectal excision for the treatment of mid and low rectal cancer: a meta-analysis. Eur J Surg Oncol 2016;42(12):1841–50.
78. Marks JH, Lopez-Acevedo N, Krishnan B, et al. True NOTES TME resection with splenic flexure release, high ligation of IMA, and side-to-end hand-sewn coloanal anastomosis. Surg Endosc 2016;30(10):4626–31.
79. Leroy J, Barry BD, Melani A, et al. No-scar transanal total mesorectal excision: the last step to pure NOTES for colorectal surgery. JAMA Surg 2013;148(3):226–30 [discussion: 231].
80. Rattner DW, Smith CD. 25(th) Anniversary state-of-the-art expert discussion with David W. Rattner, MD, on NOTES. J Laparoendosc Adv Surg Tech A 2015;25(12): 961–5.
81. Hawes RH. Lessons learned from traditional NOTES: a historical perspective [review]. Gastrointest Endosc Clin N Am 2016;26(2):221–7.
82. Borstlap WA, Tanis PJ, Koedam TW, et al. A multi-centred randomised trial of radical surgery versus adjuvant chemoradiotherapy after local excision for early rectal cancer. BMC Cancer 2016;16:513.
83. Serra-Aracil X, Pericay C, Golda T, et al. TAU-TEM study group. Non-inferiority multicenter prospective randomized controlled study of rectal cancer T_2-T_{3s}(superficial) N_0, M_0 undergoing neoadjuvant treatment and local excision (TEM) vs total mesorectal excision (TME). Int J Colorectal Dis 2018;33(2):241–9.
84. Rombouts AJM, Al-Najami I, Abbott NL, et al, for STAR-TREC Collaborative Group. Can we Save the rectum by watchful waiting or TransAnal microsurgery following (chemo) Radiotherapy versus Total mesorectal excision for early REctal Cancer (STAR-TREC study)?: protocol for a multicentre, randomised feasibility study. BMJ Open 2017;7(12):e019474.
85. Simillis C, Hompes R, Penna M, et al. A systematic review of transanal total mesorectal excision: is this the future of rectal cancer surgery? Colorectal Dis 2016; 18(1):19–36.

86. Atallah S. Transanal minimally invasive surgery for total mesorectal excision. Minim Invasive Ther Allied Technol 2014;23(1):10–6.
87. Francis N, Penna M, Mackenzie H, et al, International TaTME Educational Collaborative Group. Consensus on structured training curriculum for transanal total mesorectal excision (TaTME). Surg Endosc 2017;31(7):2711–9.
88. McLemore EC, Harnsberger CR, Broderick RC, et al. Transanal total mesorectal excision (taTME) for rectal cancer: a training pathway. Surg Endosc 2016;30(9): 4130–5.
89. Adamina M, Buchs NC, Penna M, et al, St. Gallen Colorectal Consensus Expert Group. St. Gallen consensus on safe implementation of transanal total mesorectal excision. Surg Endosc 2018;32(3):1091–103.
90. Deijen CL, Velthuis S, Tsai A, et al. COLOR III: a multicentre randomised clinical trial comparing transanal TME versus laparoscopic TME for mid and low rectal cancer. Surg Endosc 2016;30(8):3210–5.

Robotic Head and Neck Surgery

Andrey Finegersh, MD[a], Floyd Christopher Holsinger, MD[b], Neil D. Gross, MD[c], Ryan K. Orosco, MD[a],*

KEYWORDS

- Transoral robotic surgery • Minimally invasive surgery • Robotic surgery
- Head and neck surgery • Transoral endoscopic head and neck surgery

KEY POINTS

- Transoral robotic surgery was developed in 2005 and has emerged over the last decade as a tool for resecting oropharyngeal, hypopharyngeal, and laryngeal tumors.
- In carefully selected patients, transaxillary, transoral, and retroauricular robotic approaches to the neck and thyroid may obviate a neck incision and have demonstrated promising oncologic and quality-of-life outcomes in some populations.
- Emerging robotic platforms use single-port access and flexible instruments to increase access to the upper aerodigestive tract.

INTRODUCTION

Since its inception, otolaryngology has been driven forward by pioneers who skillfully adapt new technologies to the intricate anatomy of the ear, nose, throat, and neck. In 1921, Carl Nylen, a Swedish Otolaryngologist, used the monocular microscope to treat chronic otitis media. The next year, Gunnar Holmgren, Nylen's chief, introduced the first binocular microscope by attaching a light source to an existing Zeiss microscope.[1] In the 1970s, Walter Messerklinger and his protégé, Heinz Stammberger in Graz Austria pioneered endoscopic sinus surgery that was later popularized and refined by David Kennedy in the United States. This pioneering work opened the minds of the next generation that led to the development and innovation of minimally invasive head and neck surgery.

Disclosure: The authors declare that there are no conflicts of interest related to this study.
[a] Head and Neck Surgical Oncology, Moores Cancer Center, University of California San Diego, 3855 Health Sciences Drive #0987, La Jolla, CA 92093-0987, USA; [b] Division of Head and Neck Surgery, Stanford University, 875 Blake Wilbur Drive, Palo Alto, CA 94305-5820, USA; [c] Department of Head and Neck Surgery, University of Texas MD Anderson Cancer Center, 1400 Pressler Street, Unit 1445, Houston, TX 77030, USA
* Corresponding author. Head and Neck Surgical Oncology, UC San Diego, Moores Cancer Center, 3855 Health Sciences Drive #0987, La Jolla, CA 92093-0987.
E-mail address: rorosco@ucsd.edu

Surg Oncol Clin N Am 28 (2019) 115–128
https://doi.org/10.1016/j.soc.2018.07.008
1055-3207/19/© 2018 Elsevier Inc. All rights reserved.
surgonc.theclinics.com

In the modern era, surgical robotics has spawned a revolution in minimally invasive surgery. In 2007, the Society of American Gastrointestinal and Endoscopic Surgeons and the Minimally invasive Robotic Association defined "robotic surgery" as "a surgical procedure or technology that adds a computer technology-enhanced device to the interaction between a surgeon and a patient during a surgical operation and assumes some degree of control heretofore completely reserved for the surgeon." In robotic surgery, the surgeon's hands are physically separated from the patient. The robotic instruments engage the patient's tissues, and the procedure is aided by a bedside surgical assistant. Surgery is performed in a virtual environment, allowing the surgeon to interact with surgical anatomy with a novel perspective, in otherwise inaccessible places with enhanced detail.

The field of robotic head and neck surgery grew out of seminal work by Hockstein and colleagues.[2–4] Today, minimally invasive transoral endoscopic head and neck surgery is now an essential aspect of surgical treatment of malignant and benign diseases.[5] Minimally invasive and robotic approaches for neck dissection and thyroid surgery have experienced several refinements. Skull base robotic surgery may see further growth with miniaturization and advances in minimally invasive platforms. Herein, the authors provide perspective on the current state of the field and offer insight into the next generation.

CURRENT APPROACHES

The surgical robot has become a prominent part of head and neck surgery, the most prominent realm being that of transoral robotic surgery (TORS). Procedure steps, patient positioning, and equipment have been refined and standardized. Currently, the da Vinci Surgical System (Intuitive Surgical Inc, Sunnyvale, CA, USA) is the most widely utilized platform for robotic surgery. The da Vinci S, Si, and Xi platforms have multiple arms based on a laparoscopic design, one arm for the binocular endoscope and additional arms deliver surgical instruments from unique trajectories. The surgeon sits in a remote console where the surgeon views the 3-dimensional anatomy and controls the instruments. An assistant surgeon sits at the head of the bed and facilitates the operation by performing suction, retraction, and countertraction, clipping vessels, and grasping specimens. The assistant watches a screen where a 2-dimensional version of the surgeon's view is displayed.

For robotic head and neck surgery, patient positioning is critical for surgical access. To achieve adequate transoral exposure, Feyh-Kastenbauer (FK), Crowe-Davis, McIvor, and Dingman retractors are commonly used. These instruments attempt to maximize space within the oral cavity for the camera and surgical instruments. There are specific positioning and access techniques for the various subsites in the head and neck, particularly for transcervical neck and thyroid procedures and in the nasopharynx and skull base.

Transoral Robotic Surgery

In 2003, McLeod and Melder[6] performed the first transoral robotic procedure, removing a vallecular cyst with the first-generation da Vinci robot and a slotted laryngoscope.[6] TORS was subsequently established by Hockstein and colleagues[2–4] in a series of landmark papers beginning in 2005. These new TORS approaches used retractors instead of laryngoscopes.

Hockstein and colleagues[7] and O'Malley and colleagues[8] demonstrated TORS in cadaver and animal models,[7,8] and then in humans.[8] These studies established the role of TORS in surgical resection of oropharyngeal tumors. Since then, multiple studies have demonstrated the feasibility of TORS for patients with head and neck cancer.

In 2009, Moore and colleagues[9] reported the first large prospective case series of 45 patients with previously untreated T1 to T4a oropharyngeal squamous cell carcinoma (OPSCC) treated with TORS and demonstrated acceptable oncologic and safety outcomes. In 2012, a multicenter study that further strengthened the feasibility, oncologic measures, and safety of TORS.[10] The technology seemed to facilitate consistent tumor resection margins (**Fig. 1**) through a natural-orifice transoral minimally invasive approach, as reliably as if performed through the more traditional open approach, which carries with significant functional morbidity.

The most common serious complication of TORS is postoperative bleeding, with most studies citing a 3% to 8% incidence. Most of these cases required take-back to the operating room for definitive control.[11–16] Notably, postoperative bleeding rates do not seem to differ between TORS and traditional surgical approaches to the oropharynx.[11] Ligation of ipsilateral external carotid artery branches has become standard with TORS oropharynx cancer resection. Although most studies do not show a difference in overall rates of postoperative bleeding with ligation, there seems to be a trend in reducing bleeding severity.[15,16]

In line with safety and feasibility outcomes, TORS oncologic parameters have compared favorably with traditional open approaches. White and colleagues[17] reported the first initial large case series on oncologic outcomes after TORS, with encouraging outcomes. A recent case series of 314 patients with OPSCC who underwent TORS demonstrated a 5-year locoregional recurrence-free survival of 92% and overall survival of 86%.[18] To date, the largest study of TORS is a worldwide multicenter review evaluating outcomes for 410 patients across 11 centers.[19] Nearly 90% of all patients undergoing TORS had OPSCC; most were staged T1-2; N0-2b. The most favorable locoregional control tended to be in patients with tumors in the lateral oropharynx.

Given the projected increase in human papillomavirus–related OPSCC, TORS will likely remain an important tool for head and neck surgeons.[19,20] Clinical trials are currently underway to study deescalation protocols for head and neck cancer using

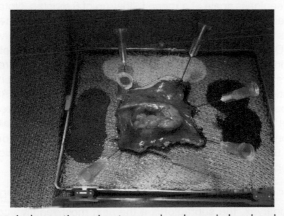

Fig. 1. En bloc surgical resection using transoral endoscopic head and neck surgery and robotics facilitates careful assessment of tumor margins. The authors recommend intraoperative assessment of superficial mucosa margins in 4 quadrants (anterior-superior, posterior-inferior, medial, and lateral) and deep muscular margins, using MarginMarker® (Vector Surgical, Waukesha, WI) to facilitate assessment with pathology." [Photo courtesy of FC Holsinger, copyright 2018.)

TORS. In July 2017, a prospective clinical trial of 519 patients with OPSCC was completed (ECOG3311) to evaluate standard versus deintensified adjuvant radiation for intermediate-risk OPSCC. In the next few years, a great deal will be learned about which patient subpopulations and which disease characteristics may be best served by TORS and deintensified treatment regimens.

TORS has also shown efficacy for identifying the primary tumor site in cases of squamous cell carcinoma (SCC) metastatic to the neck with unknown primary. A multicenter study led by Mendez from the University of Washington demonstrated the use of TORS permitted surgeons to localize the primary 72% of the time,[21] and a follow-up study by Geltzeiler and colleagues[22] found a similar rate. Most importantly, this approach may help to deescalate both the radiation dose and the field size for the previously unknown primary tumor. Patel and colleagues[21] found that several patients could avoid adjuvant therapy altogether, and many others had both volume and dose reduction of radiation to the primary site. Importantly, this TORS approach has been shown to be cost-effective.[23]

Transoral Robotic Surgery and Sleep Surgery

Obstructive sleep apnea (OSA) has high prevalence, affecting 3% to 7% of the adult population, and is an independent risk factor for hypertension, myocardial infarction, and stroke.[24] Although continuous positive airway pressure (CPAP) is effective in reducing complications of OSA, some patients are unable to tolerate wearing a CPAP mask or have continued apneas despite therapy. Sleep surgery can improve both CPAP compliance and quality of life in patients with OSA.[25] The goal of sleep surgery is to correct airway obstruction, which can be done through multiple approaches tailored to the patient's anatomy. TORS can be applied to patients with prominent or redundant pharyngeal or lymphoid tissue contributing to obstruction.

Vicini and colleagues[26] reported a case series of 20 patients who underwent TORS tongue base resection for management of OSA, with no serious perioperative complications. A 30° endoscope was to visualize the tongue base, and a piecemeal resection was performed to avoided neurovascular injury. Average preoperative apnea hypopnea index (AHI) was 36.3 and postoperative was 16.3 with a mean 5-point reduction in the Epworth sleepiness scale at a mean follow-up of 6 months. Notably, all patients underwent tracheostomy at time of surgery, and all were decannulated by postoperative day 13. This study demonstrated both the feasibility and effectiveness of TORS for patients with OSA and tongue base hypertrophy. Friedman and colleagues[27] replicated these findings without performing tracheostomy and compared outcomes to matched patients undergoing radiofrequency ablation and coblation of the tongue base. The investigators included 40 patients who underwent TORS tongue base reduction and found TORS to have a superior cure rate, greater reduction in AHI, and improvement in minimum oxygen saturation compared with radiofrequency ablation and coblation. Other groups have combined base of tongue reduction with epiglottoplasty or uvulopalatopharyngoplasty with similarly efficacious results for treatment of sleep apnea.[28]

Transoral Robotic Surgery for Laryngeal and Hypopharyngeal Surgery

Beyond the oropharynx, the supraglottis it the next most-readily accessible region. Although this area is subject to more constraints on space and maneuverability, there has been a steady progression of innovation. In 2007, Weinstein and colleagues[29] published a series of 3 patients with T2-T3 supraglottic SCC who underwent TORS supraglottic laryngectomy (SGL) following up on earlier canine model work.[30] They used a 30° endoscope and FK retractor for exposure. Ozer and colleagues[31] reported a prospective case series of functional outcomes on 13 patients undergoing TORS-SGL at a single institution. Outcomes were generally good, with 11 of 13 patients tolerating a diet on postoperative day 1 and a single patient requiring a tracheostomy and G-tube. Mendelsohn and colleagues[32] reported oncologic outcomes for 18 patients undergoing TORS-SGL. There were no local recurrences, and disease-specific survival was 100% at 2 years. Although supraglottic TORS may be technically more challenging than TORS for oropharyngeal tumors, these studies demonstrated excellent functional and oncologic outcomes.

Early stage (T1 and T2) glottic carcinomas can be managed with minimally invasive surgical approaches, including transoral laser microsurgery (TLM), with good oncologic outcomes.[33] TLM approaches rely on slotted laryngoscopes that limit exposure and access of surgical instruments, especially at the anterior commissure. TORS approaches may offer some advantages. In 2006, O'Malley and colleagues[34] described the first TORS glottic microsurgery using a canine model. An acceptable safety profile was reported with first series of 3 patients undergoing TORS-glottic microsurgery for T1 and T2 SCC.[35] Acceptable oncologic and functional outcomes were reported in a subsequent series of 13 patients with T1 or T2 glottic SCC.[36] TORS vocal fold microsurgery has been slower to develop due to technical challenges of exposure and robotic maneuverability coupled with excellent functional and oncologic outcomes with TLM and traditional laryngology techniques.

Endoscopic approaches to the hypopharynx are particularly constrained, and TORS may offer an advantage over TLM in providing access to this anatomic space. In patients with hypopharyngeal recurrence after radiation, surgical salvage has traditionally been limited to total laryngopharyngectomy, which has significant morbidity and impact on quality of life. In 2013, Park and colleagues[37] compared oncologic and functional outcomes in 56 patients with hypopharyngeal SCC: 30 who underwent TORS hypopharyngectomy and 26 who underwent a standard open approach. There was no significant difference in overall and disease-specific survival between the groups at 3 years. Functional outcomes, including quality-of-life measures, were significantly better in the TORS group compared with the open surgery group. Although these results of TORS hypopharyngeal resection are promising, experience is lacking, and TORS hypopharyngectomy has not been practiced widely.

Total laryngectomy (TL) is also possible with a combined transcervical TORS approach. Lawson and colleagues[38] reported the first TORS-TL protocol, using a cervical incision for tracheal transection and transoral approach for laryngectomy and specimen delivery. A similar approach was used in 3 patients: one patient required conversion to an open approach and another developed a postoperative pharyngeal bleed requiring take-back to the operating room.[39] Some additional case series have had outcomes in line with open TL approaches. Krishnan and Krishnan[40] reported on a series of 5 cases of TORS-TL with no significant perioperative morbidity. Chan and colleagues[41] reported a total laryngopharyngectomy with free flap reconstruction in a patient with a recurrent hypopharyngeal SCC, demonstrating feasibility of both resection and microvascular reconstructions using TORS. Additional studies are needed to establish the oncologic and functional outcomes as well as cost-effectiveness of TORS-TL.

Robotic Neck Surgery

Cervical lymphadenectomy (neck dissection) has undergone significant refinements from radical neck dissection to functional neck dissection and modified radical (MRND) approaches that leave vital structures intact without compromising oncologic outcomes. Robotic approaches to the neck follow sound oncologic principles while using novel approaches. Most of these use retroauricular approaches to the deep neck compartments, but transaxillary and even transoral approaches are also described.

The lateral neck is accessible with traditional surgical instruments via retroauricular incisions, and several studies report "endoscopic-assisted" approaches to the medial and inferior nodal compartments. Werner and colleagues[42] described endoscopic-assisted sentinel lymph node biopsy for management of the N0 neck in patients with aerodigestive tract SCC. Melvin and colleagues[43] subsequently described endoscopic-assisted MRND of levels I–V using a facelift approach. Tae and colleagues[44] reported a similar retroauricular approach in a series of 30 patients undergoing MRND using the da Vinci system.

Transaxillary approaches for dissection of levels II–V have also emerged. In a study of patients undergoing robotic transaxillary MRND for papillary thyroid cancer, Kim and colleagues[45] showed similar 5-year recurrence rates compared with conventional open MRND. Notably, transaxillary approaches to neck dissection are limited in their ability to access level I and IIb,[46] so that they are generally not feasible for patients with SCC. Combination approaches using combined transaxillary and retroauricular approaches have been developed by Kim and colleagues[47] with effective dissection and low complication rates. Most of these studies have focused on papillary thyroid cancer, where oncologic outcomes appear similar to open approaches. Several groups have proposed modifying robotic-assisted approaches by subsite for SCC,[48] with retroauricular approaches for dissections requiring access to level I; however, only a small number of patients with SCC undergoing robotic-assisted neck dissections have had oncologic outcomes reported.

Robotic surgery also has potential to access retropharyngeal nodes. Transoral endoscopic retropharyngeal lymph node dissection offers a minimally invasive approach to this space with minimal morbidity.[49,50] Troob and colleagues[50] reported a series of 30 patients with oropharyngeal SCC undergoing transoral robotic retropharyngeal lymph node dissection, wherein 6 patients were discovered to harbor metastasis to retropharyngeal nodes, and 1 patient had adjuvant treatment recommendations altered based on pathology. Givi and colleagues[51] reported a higher incidence of patients with aspiration pneumonitis after undergoing TORS retropharyngeal lymph node dissection. Therefore, although promising, additional studies are needed to explore safety, cost-effectiveness, patient selection, and oncologic outcomes.

Nearly 100,000 thyroidectomies are performed yearly in the United States, and this number is increasing.[52] Although thyroidectomy is a safe, effective procedure, traditional approaches create scars that can affect quality of life.[53] Minimally invasive approaches to the thyroid have been developed to circumvent a visible neck incision. These approaches have been popularized by pioneers in Asia but have largely fallen out of favor within the United States.

Gagner[54] described the first endoscopic approach to the parathyroid, using trocars to insert 5-mm laparoscopic instruments between the platysma and strap muscles and the operative space maintained with CO_2 insufflation.[54] Subsequent advances involved minimally invasive video-assisted thyroidectomy in which the thyroid gland is removed with or without insufflation via cervical, axillary, or anterior chest wall approaches. Ikeda and colleagues[55,56] described the first endoscopic transaxillary thyroidectomy and reported an initial case series in 2002 of 26 patients without serious complications. Although early approaches used laparoscopic instruments, this method was quickly adapted to a robotic platform. A series of 338 transaxillary robotic thyroidectomy patients showed minimal complications and excellent cosmetic results.[57] Terris and Singer[58] demonstrated the use of robotic-assisted thyroidectomy via a facelift incision. In 2014, Lang and colleagues[59] conducted a meta-analysis comparing 839 patients undergoing robotic thyroidectomy and 1536 patients undergoing conventional open thyroidectomy, finding comparable rates of permanent complications and overall morbidity; however, robotic approaches were associated with increased operative time, longer hospital stay, and higher rate of transient recurrent laryngeal nerve injuries. The American Thyroid Association released a statement supporting its role in centers with a high volume of robotic surgery for select patients with thin body habitus, smaller nodules (<3 cm), smaller thyroid lobes (<6 cm), no evidence of extrathyroidal extension of thyroid cancer, and no prior neck surgeries.[60]

Recently, transoral thyroidectomy approaches have been reported and gained popularity. Witzel and colleagues[61] reported the first cadaver and animal models for a sublingual approach to the thyroid. Several other preclinical studies were reported before the first published series by Karakas and colleagues[62] of 2 patients who underwent transoral parathyroidectomy using laparoscopic instruments through the floor of the mouth. Richmon and colleagues[63] modified this approach in a preclinical cadaver model, using an incision in the vestibule rather than the floor of the mouth. Larger case series of transoral endoscopic thyroidectomy through a vestibular approach (TOETVA) are now being reported. Anuwong and colleagues[64] recently reported a consecutive series of 200 patients undergoing TOETVA, with no permanent recurrent laryngeal nerve injuries, although 3 patients experienced mental nerve injury. Robotic approaches have yielded similar results compared with endoscopic-assisted transoral approaches.[65]

Robotic Skull Base Surgery

Accessing the anterior skull base with conventional techniques requires a transfacial approach. Minimally invasive techniques avoid open surgery in exchange for challenging exposure, visualization, and instrument maneuvering. In 2007, Hanna and colleagues[66] published on robotic-assisted anterior and central skull base surgery using a cadaver model. Bilateral sublabial incisions and Caldwell-Luc antrostomies with a posterior septectomy were used for access. They were able to place a 5-mm endoscopic and robotic surgical arm for 2-handed surgery, specifically citing this advantage for closure of dural defects. Several other investigators reported preclinical studies, including robotic-assisted suture based reconstruction of dural defects[67] as well as approaches to the nasopharynx,[68,69] pituitary,[70] and infratemporal fossa.[71] However, clinical studies have been slower to develop due to size and movement constraints of robotic instrumentation for accessing the anterior skull base.

O'Malley and Weinstein[72] described the first TORS resection of tumors of the parapharyngeal space and infratemporal fossa. The robotic approach afforded adequate and safe identification of the internal carotid artery and cranial nerves. Subsequent work further demonstrated the capability of TORS resection for parapharyngeal space tumors,[73] although this technique may lead to tumor spillage in some cases.[74] Additional studies are necessary to establish the techniques and role of TORS for resection of parapharyngeal space tumors.

Early preclinical studies of approaching the midline anterior skull base with TORS were met with challenges. In 2010, O'Malley and Weinstein reported being unable to access the midline skull base transorally using a cadaver model and developed a combined transcervical-transoral robotic approach whereby 2 trocars were inserted through the neck and the endoscope was inserted transorally.[75] McCool and colleagues[76] also described a combined transcervical-transoral infratemporal fossa in a cadaver model. Recently, Chauvet and colleagues[77] described the first clinical study of TORS-assisted resection of sellar masses. They described 4 surgeries that used the da Vinci Si system with a 30° endoscope and 2-surgeon approach. Smaller, more flexible, and multiport instrumentation is currently being developed to improve access to the skull base.

Because of the challenges in accessing and manipulating the anatomy in the naso-pharynx and skull base, nasopharyngeal carcinoma is typically treated with radiation-based regimens. Surgical salvage for recurrence oftentimes necessitates an open trans-facial approach. In 2008, Ozer and colleagues described multiple robotic approaches for nasopharyngectomy in cadaver models. They thought the transpalatal approach was the best compromise of visualization and instrumentation for the nasopharynx, cli-vus, and anterior skull base. Wei and Ho[69] described the first robotic nasopharyngec-tomy in a patient with recurrent T1 nasopharyngeal carcinoma; the investigators used a soft palate split with a transoral 0° endoscope and Dingman retractor. In 2015, Tsang and colleagues[78] reported 86% 2-year local control in12 cases of salvage nasopharyng-ectomy with a similar approach. Still, application of surgical robotics to nasopharyngec-tomy has remained slow due to limitations with current instrumentation.

FUTURE APPROACHES

The future of surgical robotics will bring smaller and more capable instruments, novel visualization enhancements, and intelligent image processing. The next generation of robotic platforms for head and neck surgery will likely incorporate both flexible stereo-endoscopes and flexible instrument systems. There are several such systems in various stages of development and utilization. One such system is the da Vinci Sp single-port system (Intuitive Surgical Inc).

The smaller spatial profile and physical flexibility of the next-generation da Vinci Sp (**Fig. 2**) and other emerging systems will create surgical possibilities in deeper sites within the upper aerodigestive tract. The fundamental design of these systems departs from a laparoscopic-based platform to a single-port access, such as was developed for single-port robotic surgery for TORS. The fully robotic da Vinci Sp system has flexible binocular stereoendoscope and 3 instrument arms that pass through a single 2.5-cm instrument port.[79] An alternative approach might be a hybrid system such as the "Flex" System (Medrobotics, Raynham, MA, USA), which uses a robotic monoc-ular camera. From this platform, the surgeon manually controls 2 wristed arms carrying surgical instruments, which are mounted alongside the camera. This config-uration also allows access to the oropharynx, hypopharynx, and larynx.[80]

The da Vinci Sp system with 3 robotic instruments is likely to alter the way that sur-geons think about TORS resection. Traditional TORS procedures are accomplished

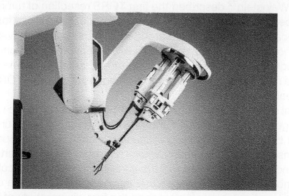

Fig. 2. Next-generation robotic surgical system using "single-port" architecture. Four instru-ments deployed from a single cannula with a diameter of 2.5 cm might facilitate innovative new approaches for the larynx, hypopharynx, and neck. (*With permission from* Intuitive Surgical, Inc, Sunnyvale, CA.)

with 2 working instruments. Early preclinical work with Sp in oropharyngectomy, tongue base resection, and nasopharyngectomy has promising results with encouraging capabilities.[79,81,82] The first 6 human cases of TORS with the da Vinci Sp have been reported.[83] Clinical trials with the Sp will continue to build on the wave of early experiences with these next-generation systems.

As discussed in the considerations for current robotic head and neck surgery, the future of this field needs innovation in the role and technique of the surgical assistant and in exposure. As surgeons access deeper parts of the head and neck, there will be a need for new bedside assistant tools. Surgeons will also need to rethink the way that the anatomy of the head and neck is exposed. Current retractors push and compress the structures that one wants manipulated surgically, there is much room for improvement. Early work in creative patient positioning for TORS tongue base surgery is an example of changing an approach to improve access.[84]

Defining how the da Vinci Sp system will fit into the practice of the robotic head and neck surgeon will take additional preclinical and early - phase clinical studies. Traditional approaches to the oropharynx will be more facile with the addition of a third instrument. The larynx will likely be more accessible with added degrees of rotation and miniaturization of surgical instruments. The challenging exposure and manipulation required for cricopharyngeal myotomy and Zenker diverticulotomy may become easier. Midline anterior skull base robotic approaches are also likely to follow, with smaller, more flexible instruments obviating transcervical approaches.

Future innovations in hardware and software are sure to push the envelope even further. Materials and mechanical engineering advances will bring stronger, more agile instrumentation. Fluorescence imaging technologies,[85] and multispectral with machine-learning image processing[86] (**Fig. 3**), will change the way that tissue interfaces are viewed and oncologic margins are detected. Semiautonomous robotic behaviors may even become interwoven with the maneuvers to streamline tasks and increase the efficiency and precision of surgeries.

SUMMARY

Minimally invasive approaches in otolaryngology–head and neck surgery are evolving to incorporate more robotic surgery approaches. The development, adoption, and ultimately, the utility of robotic approaches, in head and neck surgery depend on multiple

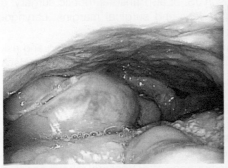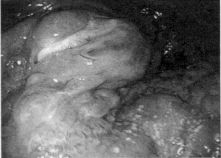

Fig. 3. Machine learning and multispectral narrow-band imaging may facilitate more precise assessment of surgical margins. The edges of the tumor on the left are less well defined in white light when compared with an examination using multispectral bands of 415-nm and 540-nm light. Both texture and entropy readily identify tumor from normal using computer vision and machine-learning algorithms. See Ref.[86] for further information.

factors: technology, safety, cost, availability, outcomes. As a new generation of surgeons receives formal training in robotic surgery, current techniques and new applications will continue to grow. In partnership with engineers, robotic platforms will continue to be improved and help push the field of minimally invasive head and neck surgery.

At any point in history, surgeons are constrained by current technological capabilities, but the future is only limited by what can be imagined as possible. In the same spirit of innovation that has driven the surgical innovators for more than a century, minimally invasive and robotic head and neck surgery will continue to grow with motivated efforts by pioneers, early adopters, and the field as a whole.

REFERENCES

1. Mudry A. The history of the microscope for use in ear surgery. Am J Otol 2000;21: 877–86.
2. Hockstein NG, Nolan JP, O'Malley B W Jr, et al. Robotic microlaryngeal surgery: a technical feasibility study using the daVinci surgical robot and an airway mannequin. Laryngoscope 2005;115:780–5.
3. Hockstein NG, Nolan JP, O'Malley BW Jr, et al. Robot-assisted pharyngeal and laryngeal microsurgery: results of robotic cadaver dissections. Laryngoscope 2005;115:1003–8.
4. Hockstein NG, Weinstein GS, O'Malley B W Jr. Maintenance of hemostasis in transoral robotic surgery. ORL J Otorhinolaryngol Relat Spec 2005;67:220–4.
5. Holsinger FC, Ferris RL. Transoral endoscopic head and neck surgery and its role within the multidisciplinary treatment paradigm of oropharynx cancer: robotics, lasers, and clinical trials. J Clin Oncol 2015;33:3285–92.
6. McLeod IK, Melder PC. Da Vinci robot-assisted excision of a vallecular cyst: a case report. Ear Nose Throat J 2005;84:170–2.
7. Hockstein NG, O'Malley BW Jr, Weinstein GS. Assessment of intraoperative safety in transoral robotic surgery. Laryngoscope 2006;116:165–8.
8. O'Malley BW Jr, Weinstein GS, Snyder W, et al. Transoral robotic surgery (TORS) for base of tongue neoplasms. Laryngoscope 2006;116:1465–72.
9. Moore EJ, Olsen KD, Kasperbauer JL. Transoral robotic surgery for oropharyngeal squamous cell carcinoma: a prospective study of feasibility and functional outcomes. Laryngoscope 2009;119:2156–64.
10. Weinstein GS, O'Malley BW Jr, Magnuson JS, et al. Transoral robotic surgery: a multicenter study to assess feasibility, safety, and surgical margins. Laryngoscope 2012;122:1701–7.
11. Pollei TR, Hinni ML, Moore EJ, et al. Analysis of postoperative bleeding and risk factors in transoral surgery of the oropharynx. JAMA Otolaryngol Head Neck Surg 2013;139:1212–8.
12. Chia SH, Gross ND, Richmon JD. Surgeon experience and complications with Transoral Robotic Surgery (TORS). Otolaryngol Head Neck Surg 2013;149: 885–92.
13. Zenga J, Suko J, Kallogjeri D, et al. Postoperative hemorrhage and hospital revisit after transoral robotic surgery. Laryngoscope 2017;127:2287–92.
14. Asher SA, White HN, Kejner AE, et al. Hemorrhage after transoral robotic-assisted surgery. Otolaryngol Head Neck Surg 2013;149:112–7.
15. Mandal R, Duvvuri U, Ferris RL, et al. Analysis of post-transoral robotic-assisted surgery hemorrhage: Frequency, outcomes, and prevention. Head Neck 2016; 38(Suppl 1):E776–82.

16. Gleysteen J, Troob S, Light T, et al. The impact of prophylactic external carotid artery ligation on postoperative bleeding after transoral robotic surgery (TORS) for oropharyngeal squamous cell carcinoma. Oral Oncol 2017;70:1–6.
17. White HN, Moore EJ, Rosenthal EL, et al. Transoral robotic-assisted surgery for head and neck squamous cell carcinoma: one- and 2-year survival analysis. Arch Otolaryngol Head Neck Surg 2010;136:1248–52.
18. Moore EJ, Van Abel KM, Price DL, et al. Transoral robotic surgery for oropharyngeal carcinoma: Surgical margins and oncologic outcomes. Head Neck 2018;40: 747–55.
19. Mork J, Lie AK, Glattre E, et al. Human papillomavirus infection as a risk factor for squamous-cell carcinoma of the head and neck. N Engl J Med 2001;344: 1125–31.
20. Pytynia KB, Dahlstrom KR, Sturgis EM. Epidemiology of HPV-associated oropharyngeal cancer. Oral Oncol 2014;50:380–6.
21. Patel SA, Parvathaneni A, Parvathaneni U, et al. Post-operative therapy following transoral robotic surgery for unknown primary cancers of the head and neck. Oral Oncol 2017;72:150–6.
22. Geltzeiler M, Doerfler S, Turner M, et al. Transoral robotic surgery for management of cervical unknown primary squamous cell carcinoma: Updates on efficacy, surgical technique and margin status. Oral Oncol 2017;66:9–13.
23. Byrd JK, Smith KJ, de Almeida JR, et al. Transoral robotic surgery and the unknown primary: a cost-effectiveness analysis. Otolaryngol Head Neck Surg 2014;150:976–82.
24. Punjabi NM. The epidemiology of adult obstructive sleep apnea. Proc Am Thorac Soc 2008;5:136–43.
25. Mehra P, Wolford LM. Surgical management of obstructive sleep apnea. Proc (Bayl Univ Med Cent) 2000;13:338–42.
26. Vicini C, Dallan I, Canzi P, et al. Transoral robotic surgery of the tongue base in obstructive sleep Apnea-Hypopnea syndrome: anatomic considerations and clinical experience. Head Neck 2012;34:15–22.
27. Friedman M, Hamilton C, Samuelson CG, et al. Transoral robotic glossectomy for the treatment of obstructive sleep apnea-hypopnea syndrome. Otolaryngol Head Neck Surg 2012;146:854–62.
28. Lin HS, Rowley JA, Folbe AJ, et al. Transoral robotic surgery for treatment of obstructive sleep apnea: factors predicting surgical response. Laryngoscope 2015;125:1013–20.
29. Weinstein GS, O'Malley BW Jr, Snyder W, et al. Transoral robotic surgery: supraglottic partial laryngectomy. Ann Otol Rhinol Laryngol 2007;116:19–23.
30. Weinstein GS, O'Malley B W Jr, Hockstein NG. Transoral robotic surgery: supraglottic laryngectomy in a canine model. Laryngoscope 2005;115:1315–9.
31. Ozer E, Alvarez B, Kakarala K, et al. Clinical outcomes of transoral robotic supraglottic laryngectomy. Head Neck 2013;35:1158–61.
32. Mendelsohn AH, Remacle M, Van Der Vorst S, et al. Outcomes following transoral robotic surgery: supraglottic laryngectomy. Laryngoscope 2013;123:208–14.
33. Ansarin M, Santoro L, Cattaneo A, et al, Laser surgery for early glottic cancer: impact of margin status on local control and organ preservation. Arch Otolaryngol Head Neck Surg 2009;135:385–90.
34. O'Malley BW, Weinstein GS, Hockstein NG. Transoral Robotic Surgery (TORS): Glottic microsurgery in a canine model. J Voice 2006;20:263–8.
35. Park YM, Lee WJ, Lee JG, et al. Transoral robotic surgery (TORS) in laryngeal and hypopharyngeal cancer. J Laparoendosc Adv Surg Tech A 2009;19:361–8.

36. Lallemant B, Chambon G, Garrel R, et al. Transoral robotic surgery for the treatment of T1-T2 carcinoma of the larynx: preliminary study. Laryngoscope 2013; 123:2485–90.
37. Park YM, Byeon HK, Chung HP, et al. Comparison study of transoral robotic surgery and radical open surgery for hypopharyngeal cancer. Acta Otolaryngol 2013;133:641–8.
38. Lawson G, Mendelsohn AH, Van Der Vorst S, et al. Transoral robotic surgery total laryngectomy. Laryngoscope 2013;123:193–6.
39. Dowthwaite S, Nichols AC, Yoo J, et al. Transoral robotic total laryngectomy: report of 3 cases. Head Neck 2013;35:E338–42.
40. Krishnan G, Krishnan S. Transoral robotic surgery total laryngectomy: evaluation of functional and survival outcomes in a retrospective case series at a single institution. ORL J Otorhinolaryngol Relat Spec 2017;79:191–201.
41. Chan JYW, Chan RCL, Chow VLY, et al. Transoral robotic total laryngopharyngectomy and free jejunal flap reconstruction for hypopharyngeal cancer. Oral Oncol 2017;72:194–6.
42. Werner JA, Sapundzhiev NR, Teymoortash A, et al. Endoscopic sentinel lymphadenectomy as a new diagnostic approach in the N0 neck. Eur Arch Otorhinolaryngol 2004;261:463–8.
43. Melvin TA, Eliades SJ, Ha PK, et al. Neck dissection through a facelift incision. Laryngoscope 2012;122:2700–6.
44. Tae K, Ji YB, Song CM, et al. Robotic selective neck dissection by a postauricular facelift approach: comparison with conventional neck dissection. Otolaryngol Head Neck Surg 2014;150:394–400.
45. Kim MJ, Lee J, Lee SG, et al. Transaxillary robotic modified radical neck dissection: a 5-year assessment of operative and oncologic outcomes. Surg Endosc 2017;31:1599–606.
46. Kang S-W, Chung WY. Transaxillary single-incision robotic neck dissection for metastatic thyroid cancer. Gland Surg 2015;4:388–96.
47. Kim WS, Lee HS, Kang SM, et al. Feasibility of robot-assisted neck dissections via a transaxillary and retroauricular ("TARA") approach in head and neck cancer: preliminary results. Ann Surg Oncol 2012;19:1009–17.
48. Byeon HK, Holsinger FC, Kim DH, et al. Feasibility of robot-assisted neck dissection followed by transoral robotic surgery. Br J Oral Maxillofac Surg 2015;53:68–73.
49. Byeon HK, Duvvuri U, Kim WS, et al. Transoral robotic retropharyngeal lymph node dissection with or without lateral oropharyngectomy. J Craniofac Surg 2013;24:1156–61.
50. Troob S, Givi B, Hodgson M, et al. Transoral robotic retropharyngeal node dissection in oropharyngeal squamous cell carcinoma: patterns of metastasis and functional outcomes. Head Neck 2017;39:1969–75.
51. Givi B, Troob SH, Stott W, et al. Transoral robotic retropharyngeal node dissection. Head Neck 2016;38(Suppl 1):E981–6.
52. Sun GH, DeMonner S, Davis MM. Epidemiological and economic trends in inpatient and outpatient thyroidectomy in the United States, 1996-2006. Thyroid 2013; 23:727–33.
53. Choi Y, Lee JH, Kim YH, et al. Impact of postthyroidectomy scar on the quality of life of thyroid cancer patients. Ann Dermatol 2014;26:693–9.
54. Gagner M. Endoscopic subtotal parathyroidectomy in patients with primary hyperparathyroidism. Br J Surg 1996;83:875.
55. Ikeda Y, Takami H, Niimi M, et al. Endoscopic thyroidectomy and parathyroidectomy by the axillary approach: a preliminary report. Surg Endosc 2002;16:92–5.

56. Ikeda Y, Takami H, Sasaki Y, et al. Endoscopic neck surgery by the axillary approach. J Am Coll Surg 2000;191:336–40.
57. Kang SW, Lee SC, Lee SH, et al. Robotic thyroid surgery using a gasless, trans-axillary approach and the da Vinci S system: the operative outcomes of 338 consecutive patients. Surgery 2009;146:1048–55.
58. Terris DJ, Singer MC. Qualitative and quantitative differences between 2 robotic thyroidectomy techniques. Otolaryngol Head Neck Surg 2012;147:20–5.
59. Lang BH, Wong CK, Tsang JS, et al. A systematic review and meta-analysis comparing surgically-related complications between robotic-assisted thyroidec-tomy and conventional open thyroidectomy. Ann Surg Oncol 2014;21:850–61.
60. Berber E, Bernet V, Fahey TJ 3rd, et al. American thyroid association statement on remote-access thyroid surgery. Thyroid 2016;26:331–7.
61. Witzel K, von Rahden BH, Kaminski C, et al. Transoral access for endoscopic thy-roid resection. Surg Endosc 2008;22:1871–5.
62. Karakas E, Steinfeldt T, Gockel A, et al. Transoral thyroid and parathyroid surgery–development of a new transoral technique. Surgery 2011;150:108–15.
63. Richmon JD, Holsinger FC, Kandil E, et al. Transoral robotic-assisted thyroidec-tomy with central neck dissection: preclinical cadaver feasibility study and pro-posed surgical technique. J Robot Surg 2011;5:279–82.
64. Anuwong A, Sasanakietkul T, Jitpratoom P, et al. Transoral endoscopic thyroidec-tomy vestibular approach (TOETVA): indications, techniques and results. Surg Endosc 2018;32:456–65.
65. Razavi CR, Khadem MGA, Fondong A, et al. Early outcomes in transoral vestib-ular thyroidectomy: Robotic versus endoscopic techniques. Head Neck 2018. https://doi.org/10.1002/hed.25323.
66. Hanna EY, Holsinger C, DeMonte F, et al. Robotic endoscopic surgery of the skull base: a novel surgical approach. Arch Otolaryngol Head Neck Surg 2007;133:1209–14.
67. Kupferman ME, Demonte F, Levine N, et al. Feasibility of a robotic surgical approach to reconstruct the skull base. Skull Base 2011;21:79–82.
68. Ozer E, Waltonen J. Transoral robotic nasopharyngectomy: a novel approach for nasopharyngeal lesions. Laryngoscope 2008;118:1613–6.
69. Wei WI, Ho WK. Transoral robotic resection of recurrent nasopharyngeal carci-noma. Laryngoscope 2010;120:2011–4.
70. Kupferman M, Demonte F, Holsinger FC, et al. Transantral robotic access to the pituitary gland. Otolaryngol Head Neck Surg 2009;141:413–5.
71. Blanco RG, Boahene K. Robotic-assisted skull base surgery: preclinical study. J Laparoendosc Adv Surg Tech A 2013;23:776–82.
72. O'Malley BW Jr, Weinstein GS. Robotic skull base surgery: preclinical investiga-tions to human clinical application. Arch Otolaryngol Head Neck Surg 2007;133:1215–9.
73. O'Malley BW Jr, Quon H, Leonhardt FD, et al. Transoral robotic surgery for para-pharyngeal space tumors. ORL J Otorhinolaryngol Relat Spec 2010;72:332–6.
74. Chan JY, Tsang RK, Eisele DW, et al. Transoral robotic surgery of the paraphar-yngeal space: a case series and systematic review. Head Neck 2015;37:293–8.
75. O'Malley BW Jr, Weinstein GS. Robotic anterior and midline skull base surgery: preclinical investigations. Int J Radiat Oncol Biol Phys 2007;69:S125–8.
76. McCool RR, Warren FM, Wiggins RH 3rd, et al. Robotic surgery of the infratem-poral fossa utilizing novel suprahyoid port. Laryngoscope 2010;120:1738–43.
77. Chauvet D, Hans S, Missistrano A, et al. Transoral robotic surgery for sellar tu-mors: first clinical study. J Neurosurg 2017;127:941–8.

78. Tsang RK, To VS, Ho AC, et al. Early results of robotic assisted nasopharyngectomy for recurrent nasopharyngeal carcinoma. Head Neck 2015;37:788–93.
79. Holsinger FC. A flexible, single-arm robotic surgical system for transoral resection of the tonsil and lateral pharyngeal wall: next-generation robotic head and neck surgery. Laryngoscope 2016;126:864–9.
80. Mattheis S, Hasskamp P, Holtmann L, et al. Flex robotic system in transoral robotic surgery: the first 40 patients. Head Neck 2017;39:471–5.
81. Chen MM, Orosco RK, Lim GC, et al. Improved transoral dissection of the tongue base with a next-generation robotic surgical system. Laryngoscope 2018;128: 78–83.
82. Tsang RK, Holsinger FC. Transoral endoscopic nasopharyngectomy with a flexible next-generation robotic surgical system. Laryngoscope 2016;126:2257–62.
83. Chan JYK, Wong EWY, Tsang RK, et al. Early results of a safety and feasibility clinical trial of a novel single-port flexible robot for transoral robotic surgery. Eur Arch Otorhinolaryngol 2017;274:3993–6.
84. Moore EJ, Van Abel KM, Olsen KD. Transoral robotic surgery in the seated position: Rethinking our operative approach. Laryngoscope 2017;127:122–6.
85. Poh CF, Anderson DW, Durham JS, et al. Fluorescence visualization-guided surgery for early-stage oral cancer. JAMA Otolaryngol Head Neck Surg 2016;142: 209–16.
86. Mascharak S, Baird BJ, Holsinger FC. Detecting oropharyngeal carcinoma using multispectral, narrow-band imaging and machine learning. Laryngoscope 2018. https://doi.org/10.1002/lary.27159.

Minimally Invasive Approaches to Pediatric Solid Tumors

Emily R. Christison-Lagay, MD[a],*, Daniel Thomas, MD[b]

KEYWORDS

- Pediatric • Minimally invasive • Laparoscopic • Tumor • Neuroblastoma • Wilms
- Thoracoscopic

KEY POINTS

- Minimally invasive surgical (MIS) approaches are being increasingly used in a wide variety of tumor types but there are no pediatric trials comparing MIS and open approaches, so great caution should be taken to ensure that oncologic principles are upheld.
- Although thoracoscopic approaches to tumor biopsy are now considered the preferred method of obtaining tissue, MIS approaches to certain tumors (eg, metastatic osteosarcoma) are contraindicated in the pediatric surgical literature.
- Challenges to MIS approaches to pediatric tumors include small working space for large tumors, the need for a large incision for extraction, that heterogeneity of tumor types defies a uniform approach, and a low case volume per tumor type for most surgeons.

INTRODUCTION

Over the past two decades, minimally invasive surgical (MIS) approaches toward oncologic resections in adults have largely supplanted open surgical approaches. Mounting evidence suggests laparoscopic, thoracoscopic, and robotic techniques are associated with decreased pain, hospital length of stay, and complication rates while achieving equivalent oncologic outcomes and long-term survival. Although the pediatric surgical community was early to adopt minimally invasive approaches to congenital and benign surgical conditions, minimally invasive approaches to the surgical management of childhood cancer have been more slowly embraced because of: (1) technical and logistical concerns based on tumor size (eg, Wilms tumor [WT]) or extent (eg, neuroblastoma); (2) clinical concerns regarding adequacy of adherence

Disclosure Statement: Neither author has any relevant disclosure.
[a] Department of Surgery, Section of Pediatric Surgery, Yale School of Medicine, PO Box 208062, New Haven, CT 06520, USA; [b] Department of Surgery, Yale School of Medicine, 330 Cedar Street, FMB 107, New Haven, CT 06520, USA
* Corresponding author.
E-mail address: Emily.christison-lagay@yale.edu

Surg Oncol Clin N Am 28 (2019) 129–146
https://doi.org/10.1016/j.soc.2018.07.005
1055-3207/19/© 2018 Elsevier Inc. All rights reserved.
surgonc.theclinics.com

to oncologic principles (preventing tumor spillage, obtaining negative margins, completing sufficient node dissection and harvest); and (3) the lack of any controlled trials comparing open and MIS approaches, MIS guidelines, or recommendations within treatment protocols in either North America or Europe.

Twenty years ago, a prospective, randomized, controlled, surgeon-directed study to evaluate the role of MIS in children with cancer was closed because of failed patient accrual.[1] Study organizers cited lack of surgical expertise with MIS procedures (39% of surgeons involved in accrual were not actively performing MIS-based approaches when the study opened) and preconceived surgeon or oncologist bias toward an open approach as reasons for failure. A decade later, the international pediatric surgical community was surveyed about their use of laparoscopy and although most surgeons were using a laparoscopic approach to such conditions as appendicitis, cholecystitis, fundoplication, and ovarian torsion, almost 90% thought a laparoscopic approach to WT was contraindicated. Only 30% would use laparoscopy for a colon resection and a mere 3% would consider laparoscopy for resection of any liver tumor (84% thought a laparoscopic approach to liver resection was contraindicated).

However, over the last decade, driven in part by the favorable adult experience and a crescendoing number of case series and retrospective reports in the pediatric surgical literature, MIS approaches are increasingly used as adjunctive or definitive surgical treatments for an ever-expanding list of pediatric tumors. Nonetheless, to date, as highlighted by a recent Cochrane review, there have been no randomized controlled trials or controlled clinical trials evaluating the role of MIS in the management of solid intrathoracic or intra-abdominal neoplasms.[2] Because of this, no definitive conclusions are drawn regarding overall survival, event-free survival, or recurrence rates in patients treated via MIS approaches and a minimally invasive approach should be selected only if the surgeon is confident the extent of resection will not substantively differ from that of an open approach.

ABDOMINAL AND RETROPERITONEAL TUMORS
Adrenal Tumors and Neuroblastoma

Although neuroblastoma is the most common adrenal tumor in the pediatric population (and the most common extracranial solid tumor malignancy in children), adrenocortical carcinomas, pheochromocytomas, adrenal adenomas, sarcomas, and other neuroblastic tumors (ganglioneuromas, ganglioneuroblastomas) can also be encountered. MIS approaches may be possible and have been described in each of these diagnoses.

Treatment of neuroblastoma is particularly challenging because of its protean biologic behavior ranging from maturation with complete regression to aggressive tumor progression poorly responsive to multiple treatment modalities. For children less than 12 months of age presenting with a tumor diameter less than 5 cm, current protocols support observation with serial ultrasounds and monitoring of catecholamines every 6 to 12 weeks for 18 months. Greater than 80% of these patients undergo spontaneous regression without surgical intervention. In older children, tumor resection is recommended either at presentation or following neoadjuvant chemotherapy based on its radiographic extension and imaging features. Neuroblastoma arising from the adrenal may be contained to that organ or have extensive extra-adrenal extension such that it encases critical vascular structures including the aorta, inferior vena cava, and renal artery and vein. These image-defined risk factors (IDRF, **Box 1**) provide objective criteria for the safety of surgical resection and the presence of one or more of IDRFs on preoperative imaging are considered to represent a relative contraindication to an

---

Box 1
Image-defined risk factors in neuroblastic tumors

Ipsilateral tumor extension within two body compartments: neck-chest, chest-abdomen, abdomen-pelvis

Neck
  Tumor encasing carotid and/or vertebral artery and/or internal jugular vein
  Tumor extending to the base of skull
  Tumor compressing the trachea

Cervicothoracic junction
  Tumor encasing brachial plexus roots
  Tumor encasing subclavian vessels and/or vertebral and/or carotid artery
  Tumor compressing the trachea

Thorax
  Tumor encasing the aorta and/or major branches
  Tumor compressing the trachea and/or principal bronchi
  Lower mediastinal tumor, infiltrating the costovertebral junction between T9 and T12

Thoracoabdominal
  Tumor encasing the aorta and/or vena cava

Abdomen/pelvis
  Tumor infiltrating the porta hepatis and/or the hepatoduodenal ligament
  Tumor encasing branches of the superior mesenteric artery at the mesenteric root
  Tumor encasing the origin of the celiac axis, and/or of the superior mesenteric artery
  Tumor invading one or both renal pedicles
  Tumor encasing the aorta and/or vena cava
  Tumor encasing the iliac vessels
  Pelvic tumor crossing the sciatic notch

Intraspinal tumor extension whatever the location provided that:
  More than one-third of the spinal canal in the axial plane is invaded and/or the perimedullary leptomeningeal spaces are not visible and/or the spinal cord signal is abnormal

Infiltration of adjacent organs/structures
  Pericardium, diaphragm, kidney, liver, duodenal-pancreatic block, and mesentery

Conditions to be recorded but not considered IDRFs
  Multifocal primary tumors
  Pleural effusion with or without malignant cells
  Ascites with or without malignant cells

Note: Encasement entails greater than 50% vessel contact and may be partial or complete.
  From Monclair T, Brodeur GM, Ambros PF. The International Neuroblastoma Risk Group (INRG) staging system: an INRG task force report. J Clin Oncol 2009;27(2):299; with permission.

MIS approach.[3–5] Case reports and small series of patients with IDRFs undergoing MIS resection have reported conversion rates of up to 50%, predominantly because of bleeding, vessel encasement by tumor, or limited visualization.[5]

When confined to the adrenal itself, without significant encroachment on adjacent organs or vital structures, a minimally invasive approach may be feasible for simultaneous diagnosis and definitive resection. In the last 5 years, there have been an increasing number of accounts of safe resection of neuroblastoma via a minimally invasive approach. Although there were initial concerns about port site metastases, these have not been reported as a complication of laparoscopic resection of abdominal neuroblastoma. Kelleher and colleagues[6] compared the outcomes of 18 children resected via an MIS approach with 61 resected via a traditional open approach and demonstrated comparable recurrence and mortality rates between the two groups. Mattioli and colleagues[7] reported on 21 patients with adrenal neuroblastoma without IDRFs resected via laparoscopy at Gaslini Children's hospital between 2008 and 2013 and compared these with 34 patients with IDRF undergoing open resection. Complete tumor excision was achieved in all patients without intraoperative complication or need for conversion to open resection. All patients who presented without IDRF (not requiring neoadjuvant chemotherapy) remained in remission at a median range of 27 months. A recent review of pediatric patients with neuroblastoma captured by the National Cancer Database found that 17% of 579 patients had a minimally invasive approach for definitive resection.[8] Compared with children undergoing open resection, these children were more likely to have a thoracic tumor, a smaller tumor, and no metastatic disease. After propensity matching, 98 children undergoing an MIS approach were compared with 196 children undergoing an open resection. Three-year overall survival was similar between the groups. There was no significant difference in margin status between the two groups. Lymph node sampling was performed more frequently in the open group (50%) than the MIS group (34%; $P = .01$) and more lymph nodes were sampled during open resections. Median length of stay was reduced (3 vs 4 days) for the MIS group ($P<.01$). Twelve percent of cases were converted from MIS to open.

For tumors that are not resectable at presentation, initial biopsy is indicated for risk stratification based on genetic classification of the tumor (N-myc amplification, 1p or 3p deletion, tumor ploidy). In these cases, a laparoscopic biopsy technique is frequently used and may be preferred over core needle biopsy on account of improved tissue yield. Laparoscopically assisted and thoracoscopically assisted core needle biopsy has also been described to assist in the diagnosis of tumors anatomically inaccessible via a percutaneous approach.[9,10]

Four principal minimally invasive approaches exist: (1) anterior laparoscopic, (2) lateral laparoscopic, (3) prone retroperitoneoscopic, and (4) lateral retroperitoneoscopic (**Fig. 1**). Which of these approaches is chosen is based on the pathology of the adrenal mass, the presence of bilaterality, and the surgeon's preference and experience level with each of the different techniques.[11,12] In a recently published European multicenter review of 68 patients undergoing adrenalectomy via a minimally invasive

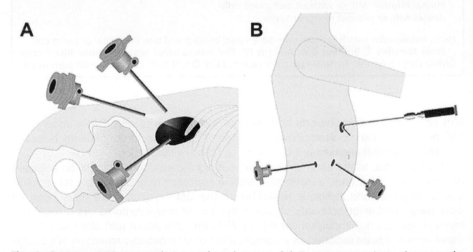

Fig. 1. Common MIS approaches to adrenal tumor. (*A*) Prone retroperitoneal approach. (*B*) Lateral transabdominal approach.

approach, however, a transperitoneal laparoscopic approach was used in greater than 90% of patients.[13] Despite its greater usage, a transperitoneal approach requires substantial mobilization of organs (colon, spleen, pancreas) to access the retroperitoneum (**Fig. 2**). Proponents of a prone retroperitoneal approach argue that access to the adrenal is facilitated by posterior-based dissection, which does not necessitate intra-abdominal organ mobilization (**Fig. 3**). Additionally, higher insufflation pressures used in a retroperitoneoscopic approach tamponade venous bleeding from small vessels. In general, tumors resected through any MIS technique tend to be smaller in size than those approached via open incisions. Relative contraindications to retroperitoneoscopic tumor resection include size larger than 5 to 7 cm (dependent on patient size) because of the reduced working space in the retroperitoneum. A retroperitoneoscopic approach typically uses three trocar sites; a laparoscopic approach uses three to five trocars sites. In both approaches the specimen is removed from the abdomen via an Endocatch bag. Conversion rates of 10% to 15% are reported. Complete tumor resection is reported in greater than 90% of cases. Surgical complication rates are equivalent to those reported with open approaches and range from 10% to 30%.[12,14–16] Regardless of the technique selected, when confronted with a pheochromocytoma or functional paraganglioma, the surgeon must make an effort to minimize direct manipulation of the tumor during dissection. Early control and ligation of the adrenal vein is recommended to limit the release of catecholamines as the tumor is removed.[17–20]

Wilms Tumor

WT is the most common renal tumor in children, with most patients diagnosed between ages 1 and 3 years.[21] Most tumors occur sporadically, although up to 10% are associated with congenital syndromes. The mainstay of treatment of WT is complete surgical resection of the tumor coupled with chemotherapy, and results in greater than 90% of patients being cured.[22] In addition to tumor histology and stage, complete oncologic resection is one of the strongest prognostic factors associated with survival in children with WT.[23] The surgical treatment of WT requires inspection of the abdominal cavity for metastatic disease, en bloc tumor resection without rupture or intra-abdominal spillage, and a regional (hilar and periaortic) lymph node resection.

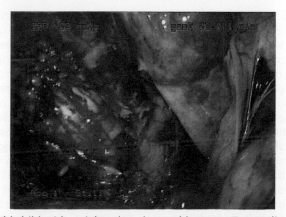

Fig. 2. A 2-year-old child with a right adrenal neuroblastoma. Tumor dissection via lateral transperitoneal approach.

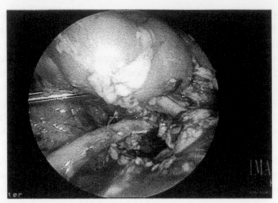

Fig. 3. Laparoscopic approach to the right kidney in patient with Denys-Drash syndrome and a WT-1 mutation.

Tumor spillage upstages the tumor is an established risk factor for locoregional recurrence and a need for subsequent radiation therapy.[24,25] Several studies have shown that the rate of tumor spillage is decreased by the use of neoadjuvant chemotherapy, a strategy used by the European trial group SIOP RTSG, but not advocated by the North American children's oncology group (COG) who argues that upfront resection of WT in most circumstances can be done safely and minimizes the chance of misdiagnosis (benign disease or different histologic subtype of a malignant tumor requiring a different type of chemotherapy) and limits the long-term side effects associated with the addition of an anthracycline-based neoadjuvant regimen.[23,26] Despite the differences in the timing of adjuvant chemotherapy, no difference in disease-free or overall survival has been demonstrated between these two regimens.[27]

Adequate sampling of local and regional lymph node basins is a requirement to complete WT staging and risk stratification; absent or inadequate lymph node biopsy may result in understaging leading to insufficient treatment and increasing the risk of local recurrence.[23,24,28] Traditional open methods of surgical resection and lymph node sampling for WT include subcostal or thoracoabdominal approaches, which optimize exposure for primary tumor resection and access to lymph node basins for biopsy.

The use of MIS for surgical management of WT is the subject of great controversy. Numerous case reports and small case series have been published claiming an MIS approach to be feasible and safe for children with WT.[27,29–33] These reports mirror the larger body of literature, which champion MIS approaches citing reduced time to postoperative mobilization and oral feeding; decreased postoperative pain; better cosmesis; and decreased risk of wound infection, dehiscence, and herniation.[30,34,35] More importantly, these authors also claim that an MIS approach is possible without violating the oncologic principles of WT resection. Nonetheless, there have been no internationally adopted guidelines regarding the indications for laparoscopic resection of WT. The lack of consensus recommendations stems from differences in treatment algorithms recommended by the two largest WT study groups: the COG WT study group (formerly the North American WT Study Group) and SIOP RTSG.[36] Because the COG recommends upfront tumor resection followed by adjuvant chemotherapy, WT specimens are often too large and too fragile (and, thus, vulnerable to spillage) to make a laparoscopic approach feasible. In contrast, tumors treated under SIOP protocols have undergone preoperative chemotherapy, reducing their size and susceptibility to rupture and allowing a MIS approach. Data from 24 children with WT in the SIOP 2001 trial demonstrated the median tumor volume regressed from 177 mL (range, 46.5–883) to 73 mL (3.8–776) after preoperative chemotherapy.[31] Neoadjuvant chemotherapy has also been shown to be associated with the formation of pseudo-capsule around the tumor.[23] Surgeons participating in SIOP protocols argue the reduction in tumor size and encapsulation induced by preoperative chemotherapy facilitates laparoscopic handling of the tumor in the abdomen, decreasing the likelihood of tumor rupture and spillage.[31] For many participants in SIOP RTSG, the question becomes whether an MIS nephrectomy or an open nephron-sparing partial nephrectomy is the preferred procedure.

Opponents of an MIS approach to WT further cite that several studies have shown that local and regional lymph node sampling in laparoscopic resection of WT is reduced compared with lymph node yield in open approaches.[8,26] Given the North American WT Study Group literature demonstrating increased incidence of tumor recurrence associated with inadequate lymph node sampling, presumably because of understaging of WT with occult metastasis, future studies of MIS resection should be directed at a better quantification of lymph node harvest. The importance of surgeon experience with WT resection and MIS in pediatric patients has not yet been studied and is likely a strong predictive factor for the successful laparoscopic resection of WT.

Overall, the limited data regarding outcomes of children undergoing MIS for WT suggest that the use of MIS is safe and feasible while adhering to the principles of oncologic resection for WT. However, most patients in North America treated under the current iteration of COG protocol are not candidates for an MIS approach. In children with smaller tumors or those undergoing nephrectomy for treatment of nephroblastomatosis, an MIS approach may be considered (see **Fig. 3**). The role of MIS will likely continue to expand within pediatric surgical oncology practice (including that for nephron-sparing partial nephrectomy), and further research will guide recommendations for patient selection and MIS techniques as surgeons gain experience with laparoscopic nephrectomy in children.

Ovary

MIS approaches that preserve ovarian parenchyma are favored in the treatment of benign adnexal masses and ovarian cysts, but there are little data supporting the use of laparoscopy in the treatment of malignant ovarian neoplasms. Despite a growing adult literature advocating laparoscopic cytoreductive surgery in early stage and advanced epithelial ovarian cancer, the Children's Oncology Group recommends an open approach to any suspected malignant neoplasms in children to ensure adequacy of resection and to reduce the chance of rupture and peritoneal contamination.[37,38] In multiple comparisons of MIS and open cystectomy for benign cysts, MIS has been associated with a significantly higher rate of cyst rupture benign.[39–41] Although there are data to suggest that cyst rupture is not associated with any increased complication rate in the management of benign cysts or even mature teratomas, tumor rupture upstages a malignant lesion. Despite these data, other authors suggest that small tumors (<7.5 cm) pose little risk for tumor spill and may be safely approached laparoscopically and removed in an Endocatch bag via small periumbilical or Pfannenstiel incision.[27]

For lesions known to be malignant, laparoscopy does have a clear role in staging. Inspection of the diaphragmatic surfaces, the contralateral ovary, and peritoneal sampling may be all be performed minimally invasively, potentially limiting the incision size require for open oophorectomy. Either single-incision laparoscopy or a more standard three-trocar technique is used.

Minimally invasive approaches can also be used for fertility preservation. Ovarian transposition and ovarial cryopreservation are accomplished laparoscopically. Because loss of ovarian function can occur with radiation doses of 4 to 20 Gy, in patients undergoing pelvic radiation at dosages of 42 to 58.4 Gy, the ovaries may be moved out of the pelvis and placed in the paracolic gutters or in-line with the iliac crests.[42] Terenziani and colleagues[43] recently published the long-term outcomes after a series of ovarian transpositions, with 12 live births in 11 patients. The only other available method of fertility preservation at the time of diagnosis in prepubertal and young adolescent girls is freezing of an ovarian cortex fragment. Although this remains the recommended practice for prepubertal girls at high risk for ovarian failure and may be accomplished laparoscopically, unfortunately, only one live birth has been reported in the literature with the use of ovarian tissue obtained in childhood.[44,45]

Pancreas

Pancreatic tumors are rare in children occurring in fewer than 1 in 500,000 children and are comprised principally of pancreatoblastoma in the infant population and solid pseudopapillary tumors (SPT) and islet cell tumors in older children. Although anecdotal case reports of successful minimally invasive resections of pancreatic lesions in children have been reported (including several isolated reports of laparoscopic pancreaticoduodenectomy and laparoscopic central pancreatectomy) there is only one larger multicenter study.[17,20,46–51] In this study, Esposito and colleagues[51] reported on the results of laparoscopic resection of 15 pancreatic tumors at six large pediatric centers over a 5-year period. Only six of the resections were for malignancy: four were insulinoma, two were SPT. Treatments included distal pancreatectomy and enucleation. There were no conversions to open resection and no early recurrences. In this series there were no reported complications, including pancreatic fistula, which is the most common complication of this procedure across all reports.[46] The authors conclude that for lesions located in the pancreatic tail, laparoscopic distal pancreatectomy with splenic preservation should be the preferred approach. However, at least one report of three children undergoing laparoscopic biopsy of SPT describes recurrences (two disseminated and one local) in all three patients at 4-year follow-up.[17] This contrasts with the low risk of recurrence or dissemination in patients undergoing open resection (typically reported about 10%) and the authors caution against using laparoscopic techniques in biopsy of SPT positing that gas insufflation may cause diffusion of tumor cells.

Liver

MIS approaches to liver resection in pediatric patients remains a nascent field with few published reports. However, the increasing use of laparoscopic approaches to liver resection in adults has provided insights and momentum to applicability within the pediatric population. Laparoscopic or laparoscopic-assisted (hybrid) liver resection in adults has been associated with decreased intraoperative blood loss and decreased length of stay when compared with open hepatectomy.[52,53] The first case series of minimally invasive liver resection for curative intent was published by Veenstra and Koffron[54] in 2016 and described the outcomes of 36 pediatric patients with 15 benign and 21 malignant (20 hepatoblastoma) conditions undergoing minimally invasive segmentectomy, sectionectomy, or hemihepatectomy. Median age of patients undergoing resection was 2.7 years (range, 9 months to 17 years). In all patients resected, intraoperative laparoscopic ultrasound was used to identify intrahepatic vascular and biliary structures and to demarcate resection margins. Division of vascular and biliary structures and parenchymal transection was accomplished by a coaptive sealing device and laparoscopic stapling. In contrast to open procedures, division of portal structures was typically performed early in the case followed by parenchymal division and finally hepatic vein division. A specimen retrieval bag was used for tumor extraction. In pure laparoscopic approaches a 12-mm umbilical port and three to four additional working ports were used. For hybrid procedures, a subxiphoid upper midline incision was used for a hand port. In this series, 31 of 36 resections including 16 hemihepatectomies were completed through a pure laparoscopic approach. Hybrid procedures were used in five cases, four of which were hemihepatectomies. Average length of stay was 3 days for segmentectomy, 4 days for sectionectomy, and 5 days for hemihepatectomy. Only minor complications (seroma, superficial port infections) were reported. All resections for malignancy had R0 margins, there was no locoregional recurrence, and one distant pulmonary metastasis in a short period (median, 12 months) of follow-up. Although this series did not incorporate contemporaneous patients undergoing open resection and reported only on a highly select group of patients chosen on imaging and clinical characteristics, it suggests that in the hands of experienced minimally invasive liver surgeons an MIS approach is feasible with good short-term outcomes and minimal morbidity. It should be noted, however, that at least one port site relapse has been described after laparoscopic resection of a hepatoblastoma with extraction through an upper midline laparotomy.[27]

Sacrococcygeal Teratoma

According the Altman classification of sacrococcygeal teratomas, these tumors range in presentation from completely external, exophytic lesions (stage I) to completely internal neoplasms undetectable by visual examination (stage IV). Sacrococcygeal teratomas invariably have a principle feeding vessel arising from the median sacral artery. A laparoscopic approach may be used to ligate this vessel before prone resection of the mass (stage I, stage II).[55,56] Alternatively, an MIS approach may be used to begin mobilization of an Altman III/IV tumor before prone removal of the mass and coccygectomy via a posterior sagittal approach.[57–59]

THORACIC TUMORS

The use of video-assisted thoracoscopy (VATS) for the resection of benign and malignant lesions of the chest has been more routinely implemented than laparoscopic approaches have been in the abdomen (**Fig. 4**). In 2010 the American Pediatric Surgical Association New Technology Committee approved the use of MIS in children with pulmonary and mediastinal neoplasms based on a review of 10 studies that evaluated MIS techniques for biopsy or resection of thoracic lesions.[60] In a recent review of children undergoing laparoscopic or thoracoscopic resection for the diagnosis or treatment of a solid malignant tumor at Children's Hospital Colorado over a 10-year period, 78 (74%) were thoracoscopic, although three-quarters of these were for biopsy and only 27% were for definitive resection.[61] Neurogenic tumors (neuroblastoma and schwannoma) and metastatic disease comprised most of these resections.

Although the advantages of a thoracoscopic approach including improved cosmesis, decreased risk of occlusis, decreased postoperative pain, and shorter hospital stay contribute to its popularity, thoracoscopy is technically challenging, particularly in infants and small children.[62,63] The tumor may be large relative to the available working space. Single lung ventilation greatly improves visualization but is difficult to achieve while compression can impair mechanical ventilation. After resection, the tumor should be placed in a specimen retrieval bag and removed via an enlarged

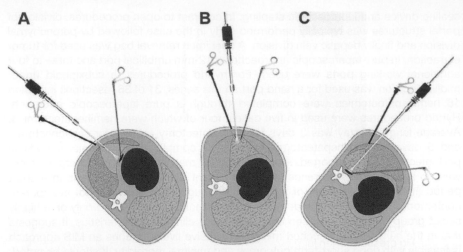

Fig. 4. Positioning for thoracoscopy. (*A*) Anterior lesions: decubitus with 30° to 45° posterior rotation. (*B*) Lung biopsy: lateral decubitus. (*C*) Posterior lesions: decubitus with 30° to 45° anterior rotation.

port site or minithoracotomy; at least one port site metastasis has been reported in a thoracoscopic resection of a neuroblastoma.[64]

Thoracic Neurogenic Tumors

Neurogenic tumors including neuroblastoma, ganglioneuroma, neurofibroma, and schwannoma are the most common primary thoracic tumors resected by an MIS approach. These tumors tend to be small and slow-growing masses located in the posterior mediastinum adjacent to the vertebral column (**Figs. 5** and **6**). There have been several case series supporting the use of minimally invasive approaches in the resection of thoracic neurogenic tumors citing comparable oncologic outcomes and similar complication rates (Horner syndrome, chylothorax) to open resection with shorter operative times, decreased intraoperative blood loss, less postoperative pain, shorter chest tube duration, and reduced length of stay.[65–67] VATS resection is typically accomplished via three to four trocars with patients in the lateral decubitus

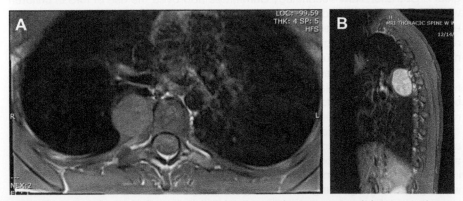

Fig. 5. (*A*) Axial MRI of heterogeneously enhancing T2 hyperintense solid paraspinal mass. (*B*) Sagittal image of same mass. There is no obvious remodeling of the neural foramen.

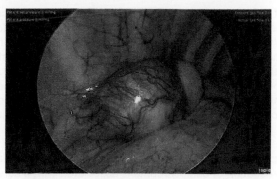

Fig. 6. Thoracoscopic view of schwannoma at T5-T6 at time of resection.

or slightly prone position using single lung ventilation when possible or insufflation to 4 to 6 mm Hg pressure when lung isolation is not possible. Although no absolute contraindication to VATS has been proposed, relative contraindications include impaired access to the thoracic cavity because of large tumor size and physiologic inability to tolerate single lung ventilation or thoracic CO_2 insufflation.

Thoracic Teratoma

Approximately 4% of germ cell tumors are located in the anterior mediastinum. Many of these lesions are mature teratomas and may be approached by MIS techniques if deemed technically feasible. The clinical biomarkers AFP and B-HCG indicate the presence of immature elements within the tumor (yolk sac or choriocarcinoma) and are markers for malignancy. Malignant teratomas tend to infiltrate adjacent structures. Because an R0 resection without tumor spillage is the most important prognostic factor for patients with immature teratomas, any consideration of a procedural approach for resection should minimize the risk for disruption of the tumor leading to local dissemination of cells and ensure negative margins. A thoracoscopic approach to these tumors should be offered only if oncologic principles can be respected.[27]

Metastatic Disease

Surgery for pulmonary metastasis was first promoted 70 years ago by the physicians and surgeons at Memorial Sloan-Kettering Cancer Center for the treatment of metastatic osteosarcoma.[68,69] In 1971, Martini and colleagues[69] at the same institution reported that 9 of 20 patients undergoing metastasectomy for osteosarcoma were alive at 3-year follow-up, a dramatic improvement from the 5% 3-year survival seen in historical control subjects. Today, metastasectomy is performed for a wide variety of tumor types: WT, colorectal adenocarcinoma, bone and soft tissue sarcoma, hepatoblastoma, and melanoma, although the evidence that curative metastasectomy confers a survival benefit in many of these tumor types is scant.

Use of VATS for the treatment of metastatic disease may be thought of either a bi opsy technique to aid in the diagnosis of a suspicious or persistent pulmonary nodule or as an excision for definitive resection. In this former scenario, VATS is the preferred approach to the lesions and is typically associated with brief hospital stays and quick recovery periods. For identification of lesions not located in the lung periphery, preoperative needle localization, nodule tattooing with methylene blue or other liquid dyes, injection of radiotracer, and thoracoscopic ultrasound have all been described.[70-73]

Survival benefit for surgical extirpation of pulmonary metastatic disease is histology (disease) dependent and may exist in the treatment of malignancies for which chemotherapy or radiotherapy is of limited benefit: adrenocortical carcinoma, alveolar soft part sarcoma, and osteosarcoma; or in cases in which oligometastatic disease responds incompletely to chemotherapy (eg, WT or hepatoblastoma).[74] Isolated case reports have reported long-term survival after surgical resection of metastatic adrenocortical carcinoma treated by formal lobectomy and wedge resection.[75,76] Provided that a resection can be performed without spillage, a thoracoscopic approach may be considered in patients with oligometastatic disease.

Osteosarcoma metastatic to the lung deserves special mention as a disease in which an MIS approach is *not indicated*. This principle has its foundation in two concepts: complete resection of osteosarcoma is associated with a survival benefit; and preoperative computed tomography (CT) is not predictive of the extent of disease found intraoperatively.[77,78] Even with modern, thin-slice CT more than a third of patients with metastatic osteosarcoma have more lesions detected at time of thoracotomy than were identified on preoperative CT.[78] These lesions are therefore treated under COG protocol by thoracotomy or sternotomy, with bilateral or staged thoracotomy advocated in some patients.

ROBOTIC SURGERY

Several studies have suggested that the major limitation to conventional MIS approaches to solid tumor resection in children are technical: limited intracorporeal space and compromised tumor exposure or visbility.[79,80] Robotic surgery offers the potential for overcoming some of these limitations offering three-dimensional views, high-definition stereoscopic optics, and improved manual dexterity along with tremor filtration and motion scaling capability.[81] Successful robotic thyroidectomy, anterior and posterior mediastinal resections, hysterectomy, cystoprostatectomy, partial and radical nephrectomy, pancreatectomy, partial gastrectomy, proctocolectomy, adrenalectomy, and oophorectomy have all been reported in the pediatric literature. However, just as with conventional MIS techniques, all data supporting its use are taken from case reports and small case series.

SUMMARY

The challenge of pediatric surgical oncology is that any given tumor neoplasm is rare and each tumor and its subtypes exhibit a distinct biologic behavior. No single center, regardless of its size or specialty, can independently treat a sufficient number of patients to make evidence-based recommendations on operative technique or surgical approach, and multicenter trials are notoriously difficult to conduct and control. Moreover, pediatric surgery already defines a subspecialty. Most pediatric surgeons have a broad surgical practice extending from congenitally acquired conditions to appendicitis, from neuroblastoma to ulcerative colitis. These surgeons may not have a specialty interest in oncology but are still responsible for the surgical care of children with cancer. Conversely, those surgeons with a dedicated interest in pediatric oncology may not be those with the most exposure to advanced laparoscopic skills, and those with the most dedicated interest in MIS may not have as thorough an understanding of tumor biology. This complex landscape of pediatric surgery and pediatric oncology provides the backdrop for all conversations about MIS approaches to tumor resection. And, because the role of surgery radicality can vary widely from biopsy alone to definitive en bloc resection with negative margins, MIS cannot be thought of as an approach with a single objective, but as a potential means to achieve a dynamic series of objectives. Nonetheless, all MIS approaches to pediatric neoplasms, whether for biopsy or definitive excision, should observe the following fundamental principles recently outlined by Fuchs,[27] a renowned pediatric surgical oncologist:

1. The operative field should be optimally exposed. Positioning of trocars is critical to exposure and also to achieving a comfortable working position. Transabdominal stay sutures should be used when appropriate to decrease the burden of retraction and spare additional port sites. Angled laparoscopes should be considered to offer a variety of perspectives and to "see around corners." When operating in the chest, the ipsilateral lung should be collapsed either by single lung ventilation, use of a bronchial blocker, or gentle insufflation of carbon dioxide.
2. Tumor dissection should procedure from peripherally to centrally, saving division of critical structures until the remainder of the tumor has been isolated. Consideration should be given to the tools of dissection in advance of the case and the surgeon should have familiarity with the use of these tools (eg, monopolar hook cautery, Ligasure, Harmonic scalpel).
3. Every attempt should be made to remove the tumor without spillage. Specimens should be placed in a retrieval bag and removed through an enlarged incision. Either a midline periumbilical or a Pfannenstiel incision may be used. Tumor morcellation should not be used because it has been associated with bag perforation and tumor dissemination.
4. The operating surgeon should have a plan in the event of intraoperative bleeding. A suction irrigator should be available. Some venous bleeding is controlled by increasing laparoscopic pressure until the vein is ligated or repaired. Ligasure, clips, endoscopic staplers, and electrocautery may all be used in the event of a bleeding vessel. Repair of a vessel with a monofilament suture may also be considered. In cases of more significant bleeding, an endoscopic peanut (Endo Peanut) may be used to apply direct pressure to the site of bleeding while a more definitive repair is accomplished.

Bolstered by increasing evidence within the adult surgical oncology community supporting MIS-assisted resections, the role of and demand for MIS approaches in pediatric tumors continues to rise even in the absence of corollary supportive evidence from high-quality pediatric trials. Although most current treatment protocols lack surgical guidelines regarding the use of MIS, the ever-growing body of case series and retrospective reviews should provide a framework for the development of multicenter trial groups, prospective registries or databases, and potentially further centralization of subspecialist services. The surgical panels of regional study groups should begin to formulate guidelines and protocols that recommend surgical approaches stratified by tumor histology, size, location, stage, resectability, and available adjuvant therapies. Until these protocols are established, MIS approaches to pediatric tumors should be viewed with circumspection and undertaken after great deliberation only if there is no reason to suspect that the oncologic and surgical outcome will not be equivalent or better than a traditional open approach to resection.

REFERENCES

1. Ehrlich PF, Newman KD, Haase GM, et al. Lessons learned from a failed multi-institutional randomized controlled study. J Pediatr Surg 2002;37(3):431–6.
2. van Dalen EC, de Lijster MS, Leijssen LG, et al. Minimally invasive surgery versus open surgery for the treatment of solid abdominal and thoracic neoplasms in children. Cochrane Database Syst Rev 2015;(1):CD008403.

3. Irtan S, Brisse HJ, Minard-Colin V, et al. Minimally invasive surgery of neuroblastic tumors in children: indications depend on anatomical location and image-defined risk factors. Pediatr Blood Cancer 2015;62(2):257–61.

4. Boutros J, Bond M, Beaudry P, et al. Case selection in minimally invasive surgical treatment of neuroblastoma. Pediatr Surg Int 2008;24(10):1177–80.

5. Tanaka Y, Kawashima H, Mori M, et al. Contraindications and image-defined risk factors in laparoscopic resection of abdominal neuroblastoma. Pediatr Surg Int 2016;32(9):845–50.

6. Kelleher CM, Smithson L, Nguyen LL, et al. Clinical outcomes in children with adrenal neuroblastoma undergoing open versus laparoscopic adrenalectomy. J Pediatr Surg 2013;48(8):1727–32.

7. Mattioli G, Avanzini S, Pini Prato A, et al. Laparoscopic resection of adrenal neuroblastoma without image-defined risk factors: a prospective study on 21 consecutive pediatric patients. Pediatr Surg Int 2014;30(4):387–94.

8. Ezekian B, Englum BR, Gulack BC, et al. Comparing oncologic outcomes after minimally invasive and open surgery for pediatric neuroblastoma and Wilms tumor. Pediatr Blood Cancer 2018;65(1).

9. Avanzini S, Faticato MG, Crocoli A, et al. Comparative retrospective study on the modalities of biopsying peripheral neuroblastic tumors: a report from the Italian Pediatric Surgical Oncology Group (GICOP). Pediatr Blood Cancer 2017;64(5).

10. Avanzini S, Faticato MG, Sementa AR, et al. Video-assisted needle core biopsy in children affected by neuroblastoma: a novel combined technique. Eur J Pediatr Surg 2017;27(2):166–70.

11. Esposito C, Giurin I, Iaquinto M, et al. Laparoscopy or retroperitoneoscopy for pediatric patients with adrenal masses? Minerva Pediatr 2015;67(6):525–8.

12. Yankovic F, Undre S, Mushtaq I. Surgical technique: retroperitoneoscopic approach for adrenal masses in children. J Pediatr Urol 2014;10(2):400.e1-2.

13. Fascetti-Leon F, Scotton G, Pio L, et al. Minimally invasive resection of adrenal masses in infants and children: results of a European multi-center survey. Surg Endosc 2017;31(11):4505–12.

14. Catellani B, Acciuffi S, Biondini D, et al. Transperitoneal laparoscopic adrenalectomy in children. JSLS 2014;18(3) [pii:e2014.00388].

15. Heloury Y, Muthucumaru M, Panabokke G, et al. Minimally invasive adrenalectomy in children. J Pediatr Surg 2012;47(2):415–21.

16. Kadamba P, Habib Z, Rossi L. Experience with laparoscopic adrenalectomy in children. J Pediatr Surg 2004;39(5):764–7.

17. Fais PO, Carricaburu E, Sarnacki S, et al. Is laparoscopic management suitable for solid pseudo-papillary tumors of the pancreas? Pediatr Surg Int 2009;25(7): 617–21.

18. Kano H, Adachi Y, Nagahama K, et al. A case of papillary cystadenoma of the epididymis mimicking a testicular tumor. Hinyokika Kiyo 2012;58(1):39–43 [in Japanese].

19. Krzystolik K, Cybulski C, Lubiński J. Hippel-Lindau disease. Neurol Neurochir Pol 1998;32(5):1119–33 [in Polish].

20. Mukherjee K, Morrow SE, Yang EY. Laparoscopic distal pancreatectomy in children: four cases and review of the literature. J Laparoendosc Adv Surg Tech A 2010;20(4):373–7.

21. Gurney JG, Severson RK, Davis S, et al. Incidence of cancer in children in the United States. Sex-, race-, and 1-year age-specific rates by histologic type. Cancer 1995;75(8):2186–95.

22. Green DM. The treatment of Wilms' tumor. Results of the National Wilms Tumor Studies. Hematol Oncol Clin North Am 1995;9:1267–74.
23. Fuchs J, Kienecker K, Furtwängler R, et al. Surgical aspects in the treatment of patients with unilateral Wilms tumor: a report from the SIOP 93-01/German society of pediatric oncology and hematology. Ann Surg 2009;249(4):666–71.
24. Shamberger RC, Guthrie KA, Ritchey ML, et al. Surgery-related factors and local recurrence of Wilms tumor in National Wilms Tumor Study 4. Ann Surg 1999; 229(2):292.
25. Gow KW, Barnhart DC, Hamilton TE, et al. Primary nephrectomy and intraoperative tumor spill: report from the Children's Oncology Group (COG) renal tumors committee. J Pediatr Surg 2013;48(1):34–8.
26. Godzinski J, van Tinteren H, de Kraker J, et al. Nephroblastoma: does the decrease in tumor volume under preoperative chemotherapy predict the lymph nodes status at surgery? Pediatr Blood Cancer 2011;57(7):1266–9.
27. Fuchs J. The role of minimally invasive surgery in pediatric solid tumors. Pediatr Surg Int 2015;31(3):213–28.
28. Ehrlich PF, Anderson JR, Ritchey ML, et al. Clinicopathologic findings predictive of relapse in children with stage III favorable-histology Wilms tumor. J Clin Oncol 2013;31(9):1196–201.
29. Varlet F, Stephan JL, Guye E, et al. Laparoscopic radical nephrectomy for unilateral renal cancer in children. Surg Laparosc Endosc Percutan Tech 2009;19(2): 148–52.
30. Varlet F, Petit T, Leclair MD, et al. Laparoscopic treatment of renal cancer in children: a multicentric study and review of oncologic and surgical complications. J Pediatr Urol 2014;10(3):500–5.
31. Warmann SW, Godzinski J, van Tinteren H, et al. Minimally invasive nephrectomy for Wilms tumors in children: data from SIOP 2001. J Pediatr Surg 2014;49(11): 1544–8.
32. Fuchs J, Luithle T, Warmann SW, et al. Laparoscopic surgery on upper urinary tract in children younger than 1 year: technical aspects and functional outcome. J Urol 2009;182(4 Suppl):1561–8.
33. Duarte RJ, Cristofani LM, Denes FT, et al. Wilms tumor: a retrospective study of 32 patients using videolaparoscopic and open approaches. Urology 2014;84(1): 191–5.
34. Jeon SH, Kwon TG, Rha KH, et al. Comparison of laparoscopic versus open radical nephrectomy for large renal tumors: a retrospective analysis of multicenter results. BJU Int 2011;107(5):817–21.
35. Blinman T, Ponsky T. Pediatric minimally invasive surgery: laparoscopy and thoracoscopy in infants and children. Pediatrics 2012;130(3):539–49.
36. Metzger ML, Dome JS. Current therapy for Wilms' tumor. Oncologist 2005;10(10): 815–26.
37. Childress KJ, Santos XM, Perez-Milicua G, et al. Intraoperative rupture of ovarian dermoid cysts in the pediatric and adolescent population: should this change your surgical management? J Pediatr Adolesc Gynecol 2017;30(6):636–40.
38. Liang H, Guo H, Zhang C, et al. Feasibility and outcome of primary laparoscopic cytoreductive surgery for advanced epithelial ovarian cancer: a comparison to laparotomic surgery in retrospective cohorts. Oncotarget 2017;8(68):113239–47.
39. Bergeron LM, Bishop KC, Hoefgen HR, et al. Surgical management of benign adnexal masses in the pediatric/adolescent population: an 11-year review. J Pediatr Adolesc Gynecol 2017;30(1):123–7.

40. Mayer JP, Bettolli M, Kolberg-Schwerdt A, et al. Laparoscopic approach to ovarian mass in children and adolescents: already a standard in therapy. J Laparoendosc Adv Surg Tech A 2009;19(Suppl 1):S111–5.

41. Tajiri T, Souzaki R, Kinoshita Y, et al. Surgical intervention strategies for pediatric ovarian tumors: experience with 60 cases at one institution. Pediatr Surg Int 2012; 28(1):27–31.

42. Peycelon M, Audry G, Irtan S. Minimally invasive surgery in childhood cancer: a challenging future. Eur J Pediatr Surg 2014;24(6):443–9.

43. Terenziani M, Piva L, Meazza C, et al. Oophoropexy: a relevant role in preservation of ovarian function after pelvic irradiation. Fertil Steril 2009;91(3):935.e15-6.

44. Demeestere I, Simon P, Dedeken L, et al. Live birth after autograft of ovarian tissue cryopreserved during childhood. Hum Reprod 2015;30(9):2107–9.

45. Guzy L, Demeestere I. Assessment of ovarian reserve and fertility preservation strategies in children treated for cancer. Minerva Ginecol 2017;69(1):57–67.

46. Petrosyan M, Franklin AL, Jackson HT, et al. Solid pancreatic pseudopapillary tumor managed laparoscopically in adolescents: a case series and review of the literature. J Laparoendosc Adv Surg Tech A 2014;24(6):440–4.

47. Senthilnathan P, Patel N, Nalankilli VP, et al. Laparoscopic pylorus preserving pancreaticoduodenectomy in paediatric age for solid pseudopapillary neoplasm of head of the pancreas: case report. Pancreatology 2014;14(6):550–2.

48. Sokolov YY, Stonogin SV, Donskoy DV, et al. Laparoscopic pancreatic resections for solid pseudopapillary tumor in children. Eur J Pediatr Surg 2009;19(6): 399–401.

49. Uchida H, Goto C, Kishimoto H, et al. Laparoscopic spleen-preserving distal pancreatectomy for solid pseudopapillary tumor with conservation of splenic vessels in a child. J Pediatr Surg 2010;45(7):1525–9.

50. Yu DC, Kozakewich HP, Perez-Atayde AR, et al. Childhood pancreatic tumors: a single institution experience. J Pediatr Surg 2009;44(12):2267–72.

51. Esposito C, De Lagausie P, Escolino M, et al. Laparoscopic resection of pancreatic tumors in children: results of a multicentric survey. J Laparoendosc Adv Surg Tech A 2017;27(5):533–8.

52. Buell JF, Cherqui D, Geller DA, et al. The international position on laparoscopic liver surgery: the Louisville Statement, 2008. Ann Surg 2009;250(5):825–30.

53. Koffron AJ, Auffenberg G, Kung R, et al. Evaluation of 300 minimally invasive liver resections at a single institution: less is more. Ann Surg 2007;246(3):385–92 [discussion: 392–4].

54. Veenstra MA, Koffron AJ. Minimally-invasive liver resection in pediatric patients: initial experience and outcomes. HPB (Oxford) 2016;18(6):518–22.

55. Bax KN, van der Zee DC. Laparoscopic ligation of the median sacral artery before excision of type I sacrococcygeal teratomas. J Pediatr Surg 2005;40(5): 885.

56. Solari V, Jawaid W, Jesudason EC. Enhancing safety of laparoscopic vascular control for neonatal sacrococcygeal teratoma. J Pediatr Surg 2011;46(5):e5–7.

57. Bax NM, van der Zee DC. The laparoscopic approach to sacrococcygeal teratomas. Surg Endosc 2004;18(1):128–30.

58. Sukhadiya MV, Das U. Laparoscopic approach to type IV sacrococcygeal teratoma in an adult. Indian J Surg 2015;77(Suppl 1):62–3.

59. Lee KH, Tam YH, Chan KW, et al. Laparoscopic-assisted excision of sacrococcygeal teratoma in children. J Laparoendosc Adv Surg Tech A 2008;18(2):296–301.

60. Gow KW, Chen MK, Barnhart D, et al. American Pediatric Surgical Association New Technology Committee review on video-assisted thoracoscopic surgery for childhood cancer. J Pediatr Surg 2010;45(11):2227–33.
61. Acker SN, Bruny JL, Garrington TP, et al. Minimally invasive surgical techniques are safe in the diagnosis and treatment of pediatric malignancies. Surg Endosc 2015;29(5):1203–8.
62. Dingemann C, Ure B, Dingemann J. Thoracoscopic procedures in pediatric surgery: what is the evidence? Eur J Pediatr Surg 2014;24(1):14–9.
63. Fuchs J, Schafbuch L, Ebinger M, et al. Minimally invasive surgery for pediatric tumors: current state of the art. Front Pediatr 2014;2:48.
64. Pentek F, Schulte JH, Schweiger B, et al. Development of port-site metastases following thoracoscopic resection of a neuroblastoma. Pediatr Blood Cancer 2016;63(1):149–51.
65. Malek MM, Mollen KP, Kane TD, et al. Thoracic neuroblastoma: a retrospective review of our institutional experience with comparison of the thoracoscopic and open approaches to resection. J Pediatr Surg 2010;45(8):1622–6.
66. Fraga JC, Rothenberg S, Kiely E, et al. Video-assisted thoracic surgery resection for pediatric mediastinal neurogenic tumors. J Pediatr Surg 2012;47(7):1349–53.
67. Malkan AD, Loh AH, Fernandez-Pineda I, et al. The role of thoracoscopic surgery in pediatric oncology. J Laparoendosc Adv Surg Tech A 2014;24(11):819–26.
68. Losty PD. Evidence-based paediatric surgical oncology. Semin Pediatr Surg 2016;25(5):333–5.
69. Martini N, Huvos AG, Miké V, et al. Multiple pulmonary resections in the treatment of osteogenic sarcoma. Ann Thorac Surg 1971;12(3):271–80.
70. Parida L, Fernandez-Pineda I, Uffman J, et al. Thoracoscopic resection of computed tomography-localized lung nodules in children. J Pediatr Surg 2013; 48(4):750–6.
71. Wada H, Anayama T, Hirohashi K, et al. Thoracoscopic ultrasonography for localization of subcentimetre lung nodules. Eur J Cardiothorac Surg 2016;49(2): 690–7.
72. Kidane B, Yasufuku K. Advances in image-guided thoracic surgery. Thorac Surg Clin 2016;26(2):129–38.
73. Müller J, Putora PM, Schneider T, et al. Handheld single photon emission computed tomography (handheld SPECT) navigated video-assisted thoracoscopic surgery of computer tomography-guided radioactively marked pulmonary lesions. Interact Cardiovasc Thorac Surg 2016;23(3):345–50.
74. Kayton ML. Pulmonary metastasectomy in pediatric patients. Thorac Surg Clin 2006;16(2):167–83, vi.
75. Appelqvist P, Kostianinen S. Multiple thoracotomy combined with chemotherapy in metastatic adrenal cortical carcinoma: a case report and review of the literature. J Surg Oncol 1983;24(1):1-4.
76. De León DD, Lange BJ, Walterhouse D, et al. Long-term (15 years) outcome in an infant with metastatic adrenocortical carcinoma. J Clin Endocrinol Metab 2002; 87(10):4452–6.
77. Kayton ML, Huvos AG, Casher J, et al. Computed tomographic scan of the chest underestimates the number of metastatic lesions in osteosarcoma. J Pediatr Surg 2000;4(1):200–6 [discussion: 200–6].
78. Heaton TE, Hammond WJ, Farber BA, et al. A 20-year retrospective analysis of CT-based pre-operative identification of pulmonary metastases in patients with osteosarcoma: a single-center review. J Pediatr Surg 2017;52(1):115–9.

79. Chan KW, Lee KH, Tam YH, et al. Minimal invasive surgery in pediatric solid tumors. J Laparoendosc Adv Surg Tech A 2007;17(6):817–20.
80. Metzelder ML, Kuebler JF, Shimotakahara A, et al. Role of diagnostic and ablative minimally invasive surgery for pediatric malignancies. Cancer 2007;109(11): 2343–8.
81. Cundy TP, Marcus HJ, Clark J, et al. Robot-assisted minimally invasive surgery for pediatric solid tumors: a systematic review of feasibility and current status. Eur J Pediatr Surg 2014;24(2):127–35.

Endoscopic Management of Pancreatic Cancer

Jeffrey H. Lee, MD, MPH[a],*, Osman Ahmed, MD[b]

KEYWORDS

- Pancreatic cancer • Endoscopy • Obstruction • Ultrasound

KEY POINTS

- Endoscopic ultrasound examination is the preferred modality for investigating pancreatic lesions owing to its high sensitivity and ability to sample tissue.
- Biliary obstructions are generally managed using endoscopic retrograde cholangiopancreatography; however, endoscopic ultrasound-guided biliary drainage is emerging as a second-line therapy in cases where endoscopic retrograde cholangiopancreatography is unsuccessful.
- Bypass surgery is generally the preferred option for duodenal strictures secondary to pancreatic cancer; however, duodenal stents remain an option for nonsurgical candidates.
- The use of drug-eluting stents and endoscopic ultrasound-guided injection therapy are still in the investigational stages, but hold promise.

INTRODUCTION

In 1985, the Gastrointestinal Tumor Study Group reported a median overall survival of 20 months for patients with pancreatic cancer who underwent surgical resection followed by combined adjuvant chemotherapy and radiation.[1] Roughly 30 years later, in 2017, the European Study Group for Pancreatic Cancer reported the results of a prospective multicenter trial comparing the efficacy of newer chemotherapy agents as adjuvant therapy in patients with pancreatic cancer who underwent resection and found a median overall survival between 25 and 28 months in all the groups.[2] Considering the survival data reflected a select group of patients who were fit to undergo resection and receive adjuvant treatment, there has not been a notable improvement in survival in pancreatic cancer over the preceding 3 decades.

Disclosure: No relevant financial disclosure or conflict of interest.
[a] Advanced Endoscopy Fellowship, Department of Gastroenterology and Hepatology, The University of Texas MD Anderson Cancer Center, Houston, TX, USA; [b] Department of Gastroenterology and Hepatology, The University of Texas MD Anderson Cancer Center, Houston, TX, USA
* Corresponding author.
E-mail address: jefflee@mdanderson.org

Surg Oncol Clin N Am 28 (2019) 147–159
https://doi.org/10.1016/j.soc.2018.07.002
1055-3207/19/

The lack of rapid improvement has many underlying reasons, ranging from a dearth of diagnostic methods, especially in early diagnosis, to poor prognostication and risk stratification, and finally to limited advances in the management of pancreatic cancer. Although the emphasis of pancreatic cancer management has generally been on surgery, radiation therapy, and chemotherapy, the lack of groundbreaking results have pushed the envelope to other modalities, both for diagnosis and management. Consequently, the ever-expanding role of endoscopy and the plethora of new tools available have led to a renewed focus on its ability to improve the care of pancreatic cancer. The arduous task of managing pancreatic cancer, now more than ever, requires a multidisciplinary approach involving surgeons, medical oncologists, radiologists, interventional radiologists, radiation oncologists, and interventional gastroenterologists. In this article, we focus on the advances in the field of endoscopy in assisting in the diagnosis and management of pancreatic cancer.

EARLY DIAGNOSIS

Despite the worldwide concerted effort to improve survival in pancreatic cancer, the 5-year survival rate remains at 6%.[3] One of the main reasons behind this near stagnant pace of improvement in survival is the failure of detecting pancreatic cancer early. Seventy-five percent of patients with pancreatic cancer present at an advanced stage where curative resection cannot be performed. Therefore, early detection is essential in improving survival. Recently, the brunt of the research in early diagnosis has been in attempting to discover a tumor biomarker. Several potential tumor markers, such as mesothelin, glypican-1, circulating microRNAs, and serum thrombospondin-1 were extensively studied, yet none of them were able to reliably predict disease. The serum protein carbohydrate antigen 19-9 is widely used but has poor sensitivity and specificity and is generally more useful in monitoring treatment response and surveillance.[4]

Although population-based mass screening programs have been successful in other tumors, most notably colon and breast cancers, they have not achieved similar results for pancreatic cancer.[5] Similarly, research into screening only high-risk groups has also not borne out any benefits. A recent multicenter, prospective trial looked at screening for high-risk individuals using a variety of diagnostic tools. A total of 225 patients who were considered to be at a high risk for developing pancreatic cancer, were enrolled; 92 patients were found to have at least 1 pancreatic abnormality (84 cystic lesions, 3 neuroendocrine tumors, and 5 dilated pancreatic duct), but no pancreatic ductal adenocarcinoma was found. Endoscopic ultrasound (EUS) examination was the diagnostic modality that found the most pancreatic abnormalities at 42.6%, whereas MRI and computed tomography (CT) scans detected only 33.3% and 11.0% of the abnormalities, respectively.[6] In another retrospective study, 86 asymptomatic high-risk individuals (carrying germline mutations in BRCA1, BRCA2, p53 [Li-Fraumeni syndrome], STK11 [Peutz-Jeghers syndrome], MSH2 [Lynch syndrome], ataxia-telangiectasia, or familial adenomatous polyposis) were screened for pancreatic cancer by EUS examination, MRI, or scanning CT over a 10-year period. EUS examination was able to detect pancreatic abnormalities in 40 of 82 cases, whereas CT scanning and MRI were able to detect abnormalities in only 8 of 82 cases and 6 of 82 cases, respectively.[7] These results have further pushed the interest in bringing EUS examination to the forefront in the diagnosis of pancreatic lesions, although widespread screening programs have not been implemented owing to the apparent lack of benefit.

DIAGNOSIS WITH ENDOSCOPIC ULTRASOUND EXAMINATION

Traditionally, most patients with a suspected pancreatic abnormality underwent cross-sectional imaging. The cross-sectional imaging studies generally included CT scans and MRI studies. The sensitivity of CT scan in detecting a pancreatic tumor varies with tumor size. Smaller tumors are difficult to detect, with a 57% sensitivity of conventional CT for detecting tumors less than 3 cm in size, and a 67% sensitivity of multidetector CT for diagnosing tumors measuring 15 mm or less.[8] Dual-phase spiral CT can detect resectable tumors with a sensitivity of 89% to 97%.[9] Although comparable with CT scanning in diagnostic accuracy, MRI has the advantage of detecting small liver metastases with greater accuracy.[10] Additionally, MRI may be able to delineate a pancreatic head mass in cases with insufficient findings on CT.[11] Although there are benefits to each, including the accessibility of CT scans and a lack of radiation for MRI studies, they inherently both have disadvantages including radiation for CT scans, cost and availability for MRIs, and the inability to obtain tissue for both.[11]

When it is advanced, pancreatic cancer is clearly visible as a discrete mass on cross-sectional imaging, in which case a tissue diagnosis is easily obtained via EUS-guided fine needle aspiration of the mass. Occasionally, however, cross-sectional imaging results are either negative or indeterminate in finding a discrete mass, and clinical suspicion of pancreatic cancer remains high. In a study by Wang and colleagues,[12] 1046 patients underwent pancreatic EUS examination for a suspected pancreatic malignancy. Of these patients, the multidetector CT findings were inconclusive in 116 patients although their clinical presentation was suspicious for pancreatic malignancy. When surgical pathology or subsequent clinical course was used as the gold standard, EUS-guided fine needle aspiration had a sensitivity, specificity, positive predictive value, and accuracy of 87.3%, 98.3%, 98.5%, and 92.1%, respectively, in diagnosing a pancreatic neoplasm in this setting. Compared with CT scanning, EUS examination was also found to be more accurate in detecting an obscure pancreatic neoplasm, especially when the tumor was smaller than 2 cm. Furthermore, the authors concluded that even when multidetector CT is indeterminate, EUS examination remains highly sensitive and accurate in detecting pancreatic neoplasms smaller than 2 cm. This property has generally led to EUS examination being the accepted modality for diagnosis of pancreatic lesions owing to its capability to characterize smaller tumors, as well as its ability to obtain tissue.[12]

DIAGNOSIS WITH ENDOSCOPIC RETROGRADE CHOLANGIOPANCREATOGRAPHY

Other conventional endoscopic diagnostic methods include endoscopic retrograde cholangiopancreatography (ERCP), and ERCP-based techniques such as probe-based confocal laser endomicroscopy (pCLE) and cholangioscopy. The benefit of ERCP is that it allows the user to obtain brushings and biopsies of a biliary stricture. Unfortunately, a recent metaanalysis showed that ERCP brushings and biopsies of a biliary stricture had a low sensitivity for obtaining tissue diagnosis, with a pooled sensitivity of 45% and 48% for brushings and intraductal biopsies, respectively.[13]

Probe-based CLE uses a thin probe with a diameter range of 240 to 600 μm that is introduced into the bile duct during ERCP. With the intravenous injection of fluorescence, the ductal mucosa can be examined in detail for malignancy. Of the features observed on pCLE, the detection of thick dark bands (>40 μm), thick white bands (>30 μm), dark clumps, visualization of the epithelium, and fluorescein leakage are indicators of a malignant process. By using these criteria, the sensitivity, specificity, positive predictive value, and negative predictive value of pCLE was found to be 100%, 71%, 91%, and 100%, respectively, whereas the diagnostic accuracy was at 93%.[14] However, this technique is novel and not widely used and most clinicians still prefer tissue diagnosis before deciding on surgical resection or initiation of chemoradiation.

Finally, in cholangioscopy, a 10F catheter (Boston Scientific, Marlborough, MA) is introduced into the bile duct through the duodenoscope during an ERCP to allow direct visualization of the bile duct. When an abnormal mucosa, polyp, ulceration, mass, or stricture is encountered, a targeted biopsy can be performed using a small biopsy forceps through the cholangioscope. However, this technique requires proficiency in ERCP and requires a dilated bile duct that can accommodate the cholangioscope.[15]

Advances in diagnostic modalities have also occurred in the field of cytopathology with the application of fluorescent in situ hybridization (FISH), a technique developed to aid in the detection of various pathologies, including malignancies, by tagging chromosomal abnormalities of interest, rendering them visually detectable. In a retrospective study of 103 patients who were evaluated for suspicious pancreatic masses, application of FISH to the tissue obtained by EUS-guided fine needle aspiration increased the sensitivity and accuracy by 8% (from 87.5% by EUS-guided fine needle aspiration cytology without FISH to 95.4% with FISH).[16]

In summary, although the use of widespread screening programs have not borne fruit, the investigation of suspicious pancreatic lesions has improved with the rapid adoption of EUS. Although other techniques including cholangioscopy and probe-based endomicroscopy are being studied, they are generally restricted to research-based adjunct modalities and have not been implemented in clinical practice.

ENDOSCOPIC MANAGEMENT OF MALIGNANT BILIARY OBSTRUCTION

One of the most common complications arising from pancreatic cancer is biliary obstruction, owing to its proximity to the common bile duct. This complication generally presents with jaundice and pruritus, but occasionally can progress to biliary sepsis secondary to cholangitis. The 2 main questions to answer in managing biliary obstruction are whether biliary drainage is necessary and, if necessary, how it should be done. The benefits of draining biliary obstruction include relief of jaundice and pruritus, enabling digestion, and avoiding hepatotoxicity of chemotherapeutic agents, but the inherent risks in biliary intervention, such as violation of sterile environment and procedure-related complications, cannot be ignored.

Over the past several decades, the paradigm in biliary drainage has shifted; endoscopic drainage has supplanted surgical and percutaneous drainage techniques, obviating the extensive recovery time of surgical choledochojejunostomy and the need for an inconvenient external biliary drainage bag. Although endoscopic biliary drainage via ERCP is safely performed in majority of the cases, procedure-related complications do occur. ERCP-related complications occur in 5% to 8% of patients and can even occur when the procedure is performed by expert hands.[17,18] Post-ERCP pancreatitis is by far the most feared and frequently occurring complication. Most patients with pancreatitis are managed as inpatients, and some cases develop severe multiorgan failure requiring admission to an intensive care unit, which leads to delays in planned surgical resection or initiation of neoadjuvant treatment.

Considering the pros and cons of biliary drainage in the context of ERCP-related complications, the question arises whether biliary drainage is always necessary. In a randomized, multicenter trial of preoperative biliary drainage with a plastic stent versus early surgery (within 1 week), serious complications were observed in 74% of patients in the biliary drainage group compared with 39% in the early surgery group.[19] However, the study was limited by a high initial ERCP failure rate (25%) and a high rate of ERCP complications (46%). Based on these data, it would be reasonable to proceed with surgery without biliary drainage if surgery is planned within 2 weeks.

For patient who will receive preoperative neoadjuvant therapy, biliary drainage is necessary. Multiple studies have confirmed that endoscopic biliary drainage with metal stents should be preferred to surgical or percutaneous drainage, or endoscopic biliary drainage with plastic stents[20,21] (**Fig. 1**). Furthermore, in patients who have undergone pancreaticoduodenectomy, the median estimated blood loss, operating time, and duration of hospital stay did not show a significant difference when biliary drainage was achieved using a metal stent versus a nonmetal stent form of relief (eg, surgery, plastic stent).[22] However, during the preoperative treatment period, a considerably higher rate of complications was noted in the plastic stent group (79%) compared with the metal stent group (7%), mainly from stent occlusion requiring additional procedures.

Metal stents can either be fully covered, partially covered, or uncovered (**Fig. 2**). A multicenter, prospective trial demonstrated increased adverse events with the use of partially covered metal stents (as opposed to uncovered stents), particularly increasing the risk of migration, leading to endoscopists generally preferring the use of uncovered biliary stents.[23] In the largest study to date comparing the outcomes between covered self-expandable metal stents and uncovered self-expandable metal stents in malignant biliary obstruction, no significant difference was found in the median overall survival and time to recurrent obstruction at 1 year. Tumor ingrowth with recurrent obstruction was more common with uncovered self-expandable metal stent, but stent migration and acute pancreatitis (6% vs 1%; $P<.001$) were seen more commonly in the covered self-expandable metal stent group.[24]

Draining a biliary obstruction by ERCP can be challenging in pancreatic cancer for various reasons. Tumor mass effect can change the angle of the bile duct and create a tight ampullary access and/or a biliary stricture, resulting in failure of cannulation by conventional ERCP. Conventional ERCP is performed by using a sphincterotome and a guidewire. To minimize the risk of pancreatitis, contrast injection is avoided

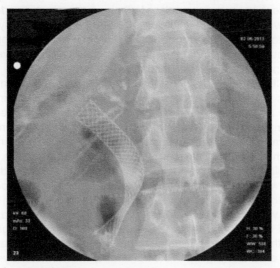

Fig. 1. Self-expanding metal stent.

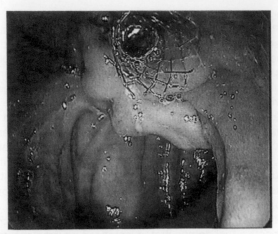

Fig. 2. Uncovered self-expanding metal stent.

by mainly using the guidewire in confirming successful cannulation into the bile duct under fluoroscopic guidance.

When there is a frequent unwanted cannulation of the pancreatic duct, a 2-wire technique can facilitate cannulation of the bile duct. In this technique, a guidewire stays in the pancreatic duct and a second wire is then introduced through the sphincterotome. The first wire placed in the pancreatic duct will block the entry of the second wire into the pancreatic duct, deflecting it to the direction of the bile duct.

In cases where the conventional and 2-wire techniques are unsuccessful, a precut needle sphincterotomy can be performed to gain access into the bile duct. In this technique, a pancreatic ductal stent can be first placed to prevent pancreatitis and help to guide the cutting direction with needle knife. Once the pancreatic ductal stent is in place, the needle-knife is advanced into the papillary os and the papilla is cut upward into the direction of the bile duct. Although it is safe and effective in an expert's hand, needle-knife sphincterotomy does require proper training and practice before becoming proficient. Improper or careless technique can result in perforation or significant bleeding, which can delay initiation of treatment. Alternatively, precut needle knife sphincterotomy can be performed from the ampullary infundibulum downward to the papillary os, stopping just before touching the papilla to prevent swelling and edema of the papilla, which can result in pancreatitis.

Although ERCP is generally considered first-line therapy in managing biliary obstruction, it is not always successful, both owing to difficulty in accessing the papilla, but also in cannulating the biliary tree. Therefore, secondary options have existed in decompressing the biliary tree. Traditionally, this was through the use of percutaneous drainage and interventional radiology; however, recently, second-line salvage therapy has mainly focused on EUS-guided biliary drainage.

EUS-guided biliary drainage generally has 3 approaches. The rendezvous method, the transluminal method (which consists of either a choledochoduodenostomy or a hepaticogastrostomy), or the antegrade method. In each method, an echoechoendo-scope is used to visualize the biliary tree and a guidewire is advanced through the use of a 19G needle (**Figs. 3** and **4**). In the rendezvous method, the guidewire is then passed through the ampulla and used as an aid to complete the remainder of the procedure similar to an ERCP (**Fig. 5**). In the transmural method, a biliary–enteric fistula is made and a stent placed in between the stomach/duodenum and the biliary tree.

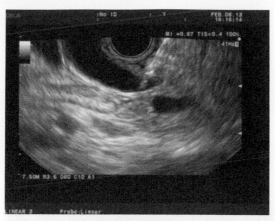

Fig. 3. Endoscopic ultrasound-guided biliary access.

Finally, in the antegrade method, the metal or plastic stent is advanced in an antegrade fashion through the ampulla (as opposed to a retrograde fashion with the use of ERCP). A recent systematic review and metaanalysis of patients undergoing EUS-guided biliary drainage after failed ERCP showed a clinical success rate (reduction in bilirubin) of 94%, although the adverse events rate was 17%.[25]

ENDOSCOPIC MANAGEMENT OF DUODENAL OBSTRUCTION

Patients with pancreatic cancer often present with nausea, vomiting, and an inability to digest oral intake. These symptoms are largely due to direct tumor invasion or tumor-related inflammation into the first and/or second portion of the duodenum, resulting in a gastric outlet obstruction. The caveat in managing a malignant gastric outlet obstruction is that the biliary obstruction needs to be first addressed, especially if considering placing a duodenal stent, because the stent will cover the ampulla and block access to the ampulla for any future endoscopic biliary therapy (**Fig. 6**).

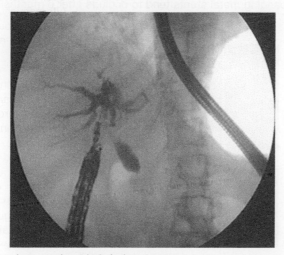

Fig. 4. Endoscopic ultrasound-guided cholangiogram.

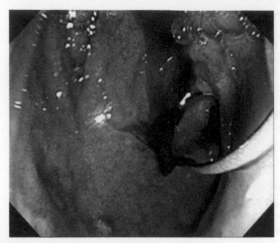

Fig. 5. Endoscopic image of endoscopic ultrasound-guided guidewire.

Generally speaking, the first-line management of a malignant gastric outlet obstruction should be surgical bypass surgery because the results are longer lasting with lower rates of reobstruction.[21,23,26] Therefore, if the patient is a surgical candidate, gastric bypass surgery should be considered instead of endoscopic placement of a duodenal stent.

Before placing a self-expanding metal stents into the duodenum, a thorough discussion should take a place among the patient, patient's family, surgeon, and all who are involved in the care of the patient because self-expanding metal stents are not retrievable and have inherent limitations and potential complications. Endoscopic placement of duodenal self-expanding metal stents is technically feasible with a high technical success rate. Before placing a self-expanding metal stent, the first step to take is to ensure airway protection because aspiration can easily occur during the procedure in the setting of gastric outlet obstruction. Other possible complications include luminal perforation and bleeding, which can occur during or after the procedure. In addition, self-expanding metal stents tend to occlude after 6 months owing to tumor

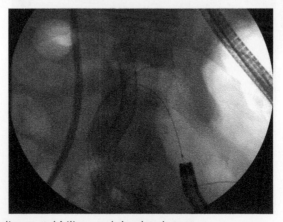

Fig. 6. Self-expanding metal biliary and duodenal stent.

in-growth through the mesh of the stent.[27] This complication can be managed by placing another self-expanding metal stent within the previously placed self-expanding metal stent (the so-called stent-in-stent placement).

ENDOSCOPIC MANAGEMENT OF POSTPANCREATICODUODENECTOMY ISSUES

Postpancreaticoduodenectomy patients can develop strictures involving the anastomosis of a gastrojejunostomy (reported in 1%–28% of patients), choledochojejunostomy (reported in 12.5% of patients), pancreaticojejunostomy (reported in 1%–26% of patients), or leak at the biliary system (reported in 2%–8% of patients).[28-32] Strictures at gastrojejunostomy sites can be endoscopically managed by balloon dilation, although this may require several sessions before reaching the desired diameter at the anastomosis. Alternatively, a fully covered self-expanding metal stent can be temporarily placed and be removed after 6 weeks. Because there is a high rate of migration with covered self-expandable metal stents in this setting, the covered self-expandable metal stent needs to be secured by endoscopic suturing on the gastric side.

The stricture at the biliary and/or pancreatic anastomosis can be managed by ERCP with balloon dilation and plastic stent placement. Although the anatomy is significantly altered after pancreaticoduodenectomy, the anastomotic site should be reached under fluoroscopic guidance using either a pediatric colonoscope, which had an ERCP success rate of 100%, or single-balloon enteroscope (or at times, double-balloon enteroscope), which had an ERCP success rate of 67% in a retrospective multicenter study.[33] One should keep in mind that there are not many accessory devices available for biliary therapy through the enteroscope and one may have to improvise at the stricture. Obviously, this technique requires proper training and experience before attempting. The most feared complication in this procedure is perforation owing to forceful advancement of the scope through multiple acute angles. Therefore, it is paramount for the endoscopist to pay special attention to how much resistance is felt as the scope is being advanced and stop the procedure, if necessary, before perforation occurs.

ENDOSCOPIC ULTRASOUND-GUIDED INJECTION THERAPY

Over the past decade, multiple small animal or human trials of EUS-guided injection therapy have been reported. The injected materials include a variety of chemotherapeutics as well as alcohol-based therapies (**Table 1**). However, it is impossible to ascertain the true impact of EUS-guided injection therapy regardless of what was injected because the patients received systemic therapy in parallel. It is unlikely there will be a prospective randomized trial comparing local injection therapy only versus systemic therapy or systemic therapy with local injection therapy. The conclusions of the studies are mainly on feasibility rather than on true survival benefit. However, the concept of increasing the drug level at the tumor site via EUS-guided injection therapy minimizing systemic toxicity can be further explored in the multidisciplinary approach until an ideal drug is found that can be locally injected resulting in improved survival.

DRUG-ELUTING BILIARY STENT

Drug-eluting biliary stents introduce 2 theoretic benefits—improving patency rate and increasing local drug level without increasing systemic toxicity. Under this hypothesis, drug-eluting stents were introduced in animal studies, with normal porcine bile ducts being histologically compared with porcine bile ducts that were treated with paclitaxel

Table 1
Use of injectable therapy in pancreatic malignancies

Author, Year	Study Type	Malignancy	Injection Therapy
Chang et al,[37] 2000	Phase I trial	Pancreatic adenocarcinoma	Cytoimplant
Hecht et al,[38] 2003	Phase I/II trial	Pancreatic adenocarcinoma	ONYX-015
Gan et al,[39] 2005	Pilot study	Cystic pancreatic lesions	Ethanol lavage
Meenan et al,[40] 2007	Early phase clinical trial	Pancreatic cancer	32P Biosilicon
DeWitt et al,[41] 2009	Randomized, double-blind study	Cystic lesions	Ethanol lavage + paclitaxel
Yang et al,[42] 2009	Prospective study	Pancreatic cancer	Ethanol
Oh et al,[43] 2011	Prospective study	Cystic lesions	Ethanol lavage + paclitaxel
Levy et al,[44] 2011	Prospective study	Pancreatic cancer	Gemcitabine
Hecht et al,[45] 2012	Phase I/II trial	Pancreatic adenocarcinoma	TNF-α
Levy et al,[46] 2012	Prospective study	PNET	Ethanol lavage
Herman et al,[47] 2013	Phase III trial	Pancreatic adenocarcinoma	TNF-α
Levy et al,[48] 2017	Prospective study	Pancreatic cancer	Gemcitabine
Nishimura et al,[49] 2017	Open-label study	Pancreatic cancer	STNM01 (double-stranded RNA oligonucleotide)

Abbreviation: PNET, pancreatic neuroendocrine tumor.

eluting metal stents.[34] Promising results in animal models led to a pilot study consisting of 21 human subjects with unresectable malignant biliary obstruction who received a metal stent covered with a paclitaxel incorporated membrane.[35] Unfortunately, their outcomes did not reveal findings as promising as the preliminary animal studies and failed to show a survival benefit compared with traditional covered/uncovered self-expanding metal stent.[36] However, drug-eluting stents had a superior patency rate to that of covered self-expandable metal stents and uncovered self-expandable metal stents (429.0 days vs 148.9 days vs 143.5 days, respectively). Although this area of investigation is fairly undeveloped, many investigators are currently working on different drugs and designs in developing drug-eluting stents.

SUMMARY

Although improving the prognosis in patients with pancreatic cancer has been fraught with difficulty and efforts to improve the outcomes in survival have met numerous obstacles over the past several decades, unceasing collaborative efforts have brought advances to translational research in early detection, accurate staging, management of the disease and its complications, and postoperative care. The incorporation of endoscopy in the algorithm of patients with pancreatic cancer has led to improved diagnostic rates and led to improvement in treating the complications related to both the disease, as well as complications from the treatment of the disease. With ever-improving tools and novel indications in the use of endoscopy, its role will assuredly continue to expand as progress is made in the care of patients with pancreatic cancer.

REFERENCES

1. Kalser MH, Ellenberg SS. Pancreatic cancer. Adjuvant combined radiation and chemotherapy following curative resection. Arch Surg 1985;120(8):899–903.
2. Neoptolemos JP, Palmer DH, Ghaneh P, et al. Comparison of adjuvant gemcitabine and capecitabine with gemcitabine monotherapy in patients with resected pancreatic cancer (ESPAC-4): a multicentre, open-label, randomised, phase 3 trial. Lancet 2017;389(10073):1011–24.
3. Ilic M, Ilic I. Epidemiology of pancreatic cancer. World J Gastroenterol 2016; 22(44):9694–705.
4. Loosen SH, Neumann UP, Trautwein C, et al. Current and future biomarkers for pancreatic adenocarcinoma. Tumour Biol 2017;39(6). 1010428317692231.
5. Pandey TS. Age appropriate screening for cancer: evidence-based practice in the United States of America. J Postgrad Med 2014;60(3):318–21.
6. Canto MI, Hruban RH, Fishman EK, et al. Frequent detection of pancreatic lesions in asymptomatic high-risk individuals. Gastroenterology 2012;142(4):795–6.
7. DaVee T, Coronel E, Papafragkakis C, et al. Pancreatic cancer screening in high-risk individuals with germline genetic mutations. Gastrointest Endosc 2018. https://doi.org/10.1016/j.gie.2017.12.019.
8. DiMagno EP, Reber HA, Tempero MA. AGA technical review on the epidemiology, diagnosis, and treatment of pancreatic ductal adenocarcinoma. Gastroenterology 1999;117(6):1464–84.
9. Wong JC, Lu DSK. Staging of pancreatic adenocarcinoma by imaging studies. Clin Gastroenterol Hepatol 2008;6(12):1301–8.
10. Sheridan MB, Ward J, Guthrie JA, et al. Dynamic contrast-enhanced MR imaging and dual-phase helical CT in the preoperative assessment of suspected pancreatic cancer: a comparative study with receiver operating characteristic analysis. AJR Am J Roentgenol 1999;173(3):583–90.
11. Semelka RC, Kelekis NL, Molina PL, et al. Pancreatic masses with inconclusive findings on spiral CT: is there a role for MRI? J Magn Reson Imaging 1996; 6(4):585–8.
12. Wang W, Shpaner A, Krishna SG, et al. Use of EUS-FNA in diagnosing pancreatic neoplasm without a definitive mass on CT. Gastrointest Endosc 2013;78(1): 73–80.
13. Navaneethan U, Njei B, Lourdusamy V, et al. Comparative effectiveness of biliary brush cytology and intraductal biopsy for detection of malignant biliary strictures: a systematic review and meta-analysis. Gastrointest Endosc 2015;81(1):168–76.
14. Caillol F, Bories E, Autret A, et al. Evaluation of pCLE in the bile duct: final results of EMID study. Surg Endosc 2015;29(9):2661–8.
15. Shah RJ. Innovations in intraductal endoscopy: cholangioscopy and pancreatoscopy. Gastrointest Endosc Clin N Am 2015;25(4):779–92.
16. Kubiliun N, Levi JU, Fan Y-S, et al. M1438: EUS Guided FNA With Rescue Fluorescence in Situ Hybridization (FISH) for the Diagnosis of Pancreatic Carcinoma. Gastrointest Endosc 2010;71(5):AB221.
17. Wang P, Li Z-S, Liu F, et al. Risk factors for ERCP-related complications: a prospective multicenter study. Am J Gastroenterol 2009;104(1):31–40.

18. Williams EJ, Taylor S, Fairclough P, et al. Risk factors for complication following ERCP; results of a large-scale, prospective multicenter study. Endoscopy 2007; 39(9):793–801.
19. van der Gaag NA, Rauws EAJ, van Eijck CHJ, et al. Preoperative biliary drainage for cancer of the head of the pancreas. N Engl J Med 2010. https://doi.org/10.1056/NEJMOA0903230.
20. Almadi MA, Barkun A, Martel M. Plastic vs. self-expandable metal stents for palliation in malignant biliary obstruction: a series of meta-analyses. Am J Gastroenterol 2017;112(2):260–73.
21. Pu LZCT, Singh R, Loong CK, et al. Malignant biliary obstruction: evidence for best practice. Gastroenterol Res Pract 2016;2016:3296801.
22. Mullen J, Lee J, Gomez H, et al. Pancreaticoduodenectomy after placement of endobiliary metal stents. J Gastrointest Surg 2005;9(8):1094–105.
23. Telford JJ, Carr-Locke DL, Baron TH, et al. A randomized trial comparing uncovered and partially covered self-expandable metal stents in the palliation of distal malignant biliary obstruction. Gastrointest Endosc 2010;72(5):907–14.
24. Lee JH, Krishna SG, Singh A, et al. Comparison of the utility of covered metal stents versus uncovered metal stents in the management of malignant biliary strictures in 749 patients. Gastrointest Endosc 2013;78(2):312–24.
25. Sharaiha RZ, Khan MA, Kamal F, et al. Efficacy and safety of EUS-guided biliary drainage in comparison with percutaneous biliary drainage when ERCP fails: a systematic review and meta-analysis. Gastrointest Endosc 2017;85(5):904–14.
26. Yoshida Y, Fukutomi A, Tanaka M, et al. Gastrojejunostomy versus duodenal stent placement for gastric outlet obstruction in patients with unresectable pancreatic cancer. Pancreatology 2017;17(6):983–9.
27. Singh A, Ross WA, Bhattacharya A, et al. Gastrojejunostomy versus enteral self-expanding metal stent placement in patients with a malignant gastric outlet obstruction. Gastrointest Interv 2013;2(2):94–8.
28. Fringeli Y, Worreth M, Langer I. Gastrojejunal anastomosis complications and their management after laparoscopic Roux-en-Y gastric bypass. J Obes 2015; 2015:1–6.
29. Malgras B, Duron S, Gaujoux S, et al. Early biliary complications following pancreaticoduodenectomy: prevalence and risk factors. HPB (Oxford) 2016;18(4):367–74.
30. Kapadia S, Pourmand K, Steiner BJ, et al. Su1399 the incidence of symptomatic pancreaticojejunal anastomotic strictures after pancreaticoduodenectomy. Gastrointest Endosc 2012;75(4):AB319.
31. Ghazanfar MA, Soonawalla Z, Silva MA, et al. Management of pancreaticojejunal strictures after pancreaticoduodenectomy: clinical experience and review of literature. ANZ J Surg 2017. https://doi.org/10.1111/ans.14073.
32. Dimou FM, Adhikari D, Mehta HB, et al. Incidence of hepaticojejunostomy stricture after hepaticojejunostomy. Surgery 2016;160(3):691–8.
33. Browne A, Kapoor S, Lewis AE, et al. Mo1418 a multicenter retrospective review of approach and outcomes of patients with post-surgical anatomy undergoing ERCP. Gastrointest Endosc 2015;81(5):AB412.
34. Lee DK, Kim HS, Kim K-S, et al. The effect on porcine bile duct of a metallic stent covered with a paclitaxel-incorporated membrane. Gastrointest Endosc 2005; 61(2):296–301.
35. Suk KT, Kim JW, Kim HS, et al. Human application of a metallic stent covered with a paclitaxel-incorporated membrane for malignant biliary obstruction: multicenter pilot study. Gastrointest Endosc 2007;66(4):798–803.

36. Wassef W, Syed I. Designer stents: are we there yet? Gastrointest Endosc 2007; 66(4):804–8.
37. Chang KJ, Nguyen PT, Thompson JA, et al. Phase I clinical trial of allogeneic mixed lymphocyte culture (cytoimplant) delivered by endoscopic ultrasound-guided fine-needle injection in patients with advanced pancreatic carcinoma. Cancer 2000;88(6):1325–35.
38. Hecht JR, Bedford R, Abbruzzese JL, et al. A phase I/II trial of intratumoral endoscopic ultrasound injection of ONYX-015 with intravenous gemcitabine in unresectable pancreatic carcinoma. Clin Cancer Res 2003;9(2):555–61.
39. Gan SI, Thompson CC, Lauwers GY, et al. Ethanol lavage of pancreatic cystic lesions: initial pilot study. Gastrointest Endosc 2005;61(6):746–52.
40. Meenan J, Mesenas S, Douglas N, et al. EUS-delivered therapy for pancreatic cancer: initial experience with targeted injection of 32P biosilicon[tm]. Gastrointest Endosc 2007;65(5):AB208.
41. DeWitt J, McGreevy K, Schmidt CM, et al. EUS-guided ethanol versus saline solution lavage for pancreatic cysts: a randomized, double-blind study. Gastrointest Endosc 2009;70(4):710–23.
42. Yang X, Ren D, Liu S, et al. EUS-guided ethanol injection for treatment of pancreatic cancer. Gastrointest Endosc 2009;69(2):S263.
43. Oh H-C, Seo DW, Song TJ, et al. Endoscopic ultrasonography-guided ethanol lavage with paclitaxel injection treats patients with pancreatic cysts. Gastroenterology 2011;140(1):172–9.
44. Levy MJ, Alberts SR, Chari ST, et al. 716 EUS guided intra-tumoral gemcitabine therapy for locally advanced and metastatic pancreatic cancer. Gastrointest Endosc 2011;73(4):AB144–5.
45. Hecht JR, Farrell JJ, Senzer N, et al. EUS or percutaneously guided intratumoral TNFerade biologic with 5-fluorouracil and radiotherapy for first-line treatment of locally advanced pancreatic cancer: a phase I/II study. Gastrointest Endosc 2012;75(2):332–8.
46. Levy MJ, Thompson GB, Topazian MD, et al. US-guided ethanol ablation of insulinomas: a new treatment option. Gastrointest Endosc 2012;75(1):200–6.
47. Herman JM, Wild AT, Wang H, et al. Randomized phase III multi-institutional study of TNFerade biologic with fluorouracil and radiotherapy for locally advanced pancreatic cancer: final results. J Clin Oncol 2013;31(7):886–94.
48. Levy MJ, Alberts SR, Bamlet WR, et al. EUS-guided fine-needle injection of gemcitabine for locally advanced and metastatic pancreatic cancer. Gastrointest Endosc 2017;86(1):161–9.
49. Nishimura M, Matsukawa M, Fujii Y, et al. Effects of EUS-guided intratumoral injection of oligonucleotide STNM01 on tumor growth, histology, and overall survival in patients with unresectable pancreatic cancer. Gastrointest Endosc 2017. https://doi.org/10.1016/J.GIE.2017.10.030.

Moving?

Make sure your subscription moves with you!

To notify us of your new address, find your **Clinics Account Number** (located on your mailing label above your name), and contact customer service at:

Email: journalscustomerservice-usa@elsevier.com

800-654-2452 (subscribers in the U.S. & Canada)
314-447-8871 (subscribers outside of the U.S. & Canada)

Fax number: 314-447-8029

Elsevier Health Sciences Division
Subscription Customer Service
3251 Riverport Lane
Maryland Heights, MO 63043

*To ensure uninterrupted delivery of your subscription, please notify us at least 4 weeks in advance of move.